# Erich Fromm

This book portrays Erich Fromm as a political theorist, despite the paucity of references to him in the field of political theory. It demonstrates how Fromm's political theory transcends the conventional disciplinary boundaries of political theory and how his distinctive psychoanalytic perspective is pivotal to comprehending the fundamental nature of fascist politics and addressing intricate sociopolitical issues such as authoritarianism and alienation. The book argues that Fromm's sociopsychoanalytic analysis, underpinned by his distinctive characterological approach to political theory, is indispensable for deciphering and effectively dealing with twenty-first century fascism, or what has been termed "postfascism". The book is accessible and comprehensive, and as such will be of great interest to students, scholars, and researchers of political theory, especially fascism and authoritarianism.

**Takamichi Sakurai** is a Senior Researcher at Keio Research Institute, Keio University SFC, Japan. Sakurai is the founding Co-Editor-in-Chief of the peer-reviewed journal *Comparative Political Theory* and a member of the Advisory Council of the Association for Global Political Thought (Harvard University). He is the author of *New Perspectives on Comparative Political Theory*.

## Political Theorists beyond the Canon

**Series Editor: Markus Pausch & Takamichi Sakurai**

The series, *Political Theorists beyond the Canon*, presents a selection of twentieth-century political thinkers who do not conform to the mainstream of political theory. However, these thinkers offer critical and contemporary perspectives on societal problems of their time that are particularly relevant for today. The series delves not only into the crux of the theorists' propositions but also explores the historical milieu and reception history of the proposed authors, elucidating their contemporary relevance. The breadth of their thought extends beyond the conventional disciplinary boundaries of political philosophy. The diversity of the theorists portrayed is also evident in the regional origins and cultural context of the theories.

For more information about this series, please visit:

**Erich Fromm**
A Political Theory of Fascism
*Takamichi Sakurai*

# Erich Fromm

## A Political Theory of Fascism

Takamichi Sakurai

Routledge
Taylor & Francis Group
LONDON AND NEW YORK

First published 2026
by Routledge
4 Park Square, Milton Park, Abingdon, Oxon OX14 4RN

and by Routledge
605 Third Avenue, New York, NY 10158

*Routledge is an imprint of the Taylor & Francis Group, an informa business*



*British Library Cataloguing-in-Publication Data*
A catalogue record for this book is available from the British Library

ISBN: 978-1-032-38932-5 (hbk)
ISBN: 978-1-032-98759-0 (pbk)
ISBN: 978-1-003-60039-8 (ebk)

DOI: 10.4324/ 9781003600398

Typeset in Sabon
by Deanta Global Publishing Services, Chennai, India

# Contents

# Preface

The seminal work *The Art of Loving* by Fromm was a source of inspiration during my undergraduate studies, marking the inception of my interest in his thought. This anecdote suggests that I am, in a sense, a prototypical Fromm reader who initiated research on Fromm with the book that articulates the notion of love as an art. The pursuit of knowledge regarding the act of love was not a priority, nor was the inability to love a source of concern. The impetus for my interest in Fromm stemmed from my admiration for his distinctive sociopsychoanalytic approach to diagnostic and remedial issues, particularly his interweaving of the concept of love with societal concerns.

It is conceivable that my perspective on the book differs from the prevailing viewpoint, which is predominantly associated with the field of normative theory. The normative relevance of Fromm's theory is undoubtedly crucially important; however, the significance of Fromm lies in its descriptive and problem-solving issues, as I will argue in the preceding chapters. This perspective may stand in contrast to the prevailing trends in current Fromm research. As a social and political theorist, however, I distance myself from highly normative themes. It is argued that moral and normative theorists and philosophers engage with these subjects, while social and political theorists are dedicated to the detection and resolution of societal problems, such as authoritarianism and fascism, which are central themes in Fromm's work.

In consideration of the prevailing state of Fromm research, it is both regrettable and disconcerting that the vast majority of the authors of the primary edited books on Fromm's theory are Anglophone scholars—a considerable number of individuals appear to be engaged in active involvement with the Fromm research circle.[1] A substantial proportion of scholars engaged in Fromm studies appear to be non-native speakers of English, hailing from both Western (including Germany) and non-Western regions.[2] Notwithstanding the potential unconsciousness of the editors and authors, this may be an overt form of exclusion. Alternatively, this phenomenon could be posited as their unconscious consideration of it as a natural consequence of Anglophone scholars' superior academic performance. As a non-Western scholar of Fromm and a comparative theorist, I herein state that it is imperative to acknowledge and address the geographically and even racially uneven distribution of scholarship in the field.

The book has received support from scholars in the social sciences and medical fields. I would like to express my gratitude to Thomas Fuchs, who oversaw my sociopsychiatric research concerning Fromm. It is noteworthy that I had the privilege of becoming acquainted with him in Heidelberg, the city where Fromm pursued his studies, and that he was honored with the Erich Fromm Prize 2023—I offer my sincerest congratulations. The book series "Political Theorists beyond the Canon" was conceptualized by Markus Pausch, to whom I extend my gratitude for his contribution to the project. It is evident that the initiative is pioneering and epochal. The completion of this book marks the inaugural title of the series, a milestone that I am pleased to announce.

Additionally, I would like to express my profound gratitude to Aakash Chakrabarty for his instrumental role in launching the book series and bringing it to fruition. It is with a sense of relief that I acknowledge the completion of the task associated with this unparalleled first title.

Earlier versions of parts of chapters 1, 2, and 4 have been published previously as "A Frommian Perspective on the Socio-Psychological Structure of Post-Fascism in Liberal Democracies" in *Distinktion*, 21, no. 2 (2020), as "The Socio-Theoretical Relevance of Erich Fromm's Psychoanalytic Conception of Narcissism: Towards a Frommian Critical Social Theory of Narcissism" in *Theoria: A Journal of Social and Political Theory*, 68, no. 166 (2021), and as "The Authoritarian Orientation in Liberal Democracies: Labor Market and Workplace Authoritarianism" in *Constellations*, 32, no. 1 (2025).

Finally, it is with great satisfaction that I can affirm my unwavering confidence in the fundamental principles of my own theoretical framework. It is important to note that the assertion regarding an inherent deficiency in social and political theory research due to an inadequate interpretation, predominantly from a hermeneutical perspective, is not endorsed. It is evident that the fundamental objective of these research endeavors is not the interpretation of a thinker's theory—researchers should disregard hermeneutical adequacy if it hinders the raison d'être of their social and political theory research. This book underscores its distinctive methodology employed in an analysis of Fromm's political theory, thereby putting forth the hypothesis that his marginalization from the academic community rather played a pivotal role in fostering his evolution as an original thinker. It is a source of pride for me that I was able to contribute to Fromm from a marginal position as well.

## Notes

1 See, e.g., Kevin Anderson and Richard Quinney (Eds.), *Erich Fromm and Critical Criminology: Beyond the Punitive Society* (Urbana and Chicago: University of Illinois Press, 2000); Joan Braune and Kieran Durkin (Eds.), *Erich Fromm's Critical Theory: Hope, Humanism, and the Future* (London: Bloomsbury Academic, 2020); Mauricio Cortina and Michael Maccoby (Eds.), *A Prophetic Analyst: Erich Fromm's Contribution to Psychoanalysis* (Northvale and London:

Jason Aronson, 1996); Joseph Fantauzzi, Maor Levitin, and Terry Maley (Eds.), *Erich Fromm and Left Strategy: New Paths Toward Radical Transformation* (Cham, Switzerland: Palgrave Macmillan, 2025); Seyed Javad Miri, Robert Lake, and Tricia M. Kress (Eds.), *Reclaiming the Sane Society: Essays on Erich Fromm's Thought* (Rotterdam: Sense Publishers, 2014). This phenomenon is exemplified even by prominent German-speaking works, such as Michael Kessler and Rainer Funk's *Erich Fromm und die Frankfurter Schule* (Tübingen: Francke Verlag, 1992), which highlight the substantial involvement of English-speaking scholars within the German academic milieu.

2 The following evidence substantiates this claim: *Fromm Forum* (English edition), Internationale Erich-Fromm-Gesellschaft e.V. (https://fromm-gesellschaft.eu/en/fromm-forum-english-edition); The Second International Erich Fromm Conference (https://efsc.ipu-berlin.de/fileadmin/downloads/abstract-band-alphabetisch-programm.pdf); The Third International Erich Fromm Research Conference (https://www.ipu-berlin.de/fileadmin/downloads/veranstaltungen/erich-fromm-fkz-web.pdf); Erich Fromm Seminar (https://efsc.ipu-berlin.de/en/news/erich-fromm-seminar)

# Introduction

## Why Fromm?

Erich Fromm (1900–80) is considered a social theorist of the revisionist school of twentieth-century psychoanalysis. Fromm is sometimes introduced as a Neo-Freudian psychoanalyst or a social psychologist, but the crux of Fromm's theoretical framework is best encapsulated by his designation as a "critical theorist."[1] In fact, Fromm occupied a pivotal role in the early Frankfurt School, a group of Jewish scholars who emerged in early twentieth-century Germany with the objective of reforming society and theory. They sought to achieve this through a social theory that simultaneously incorporated Freudian psychoanalysis and Marxian dialectical critique, a synthesis now recognized as "critical theory." Fromm's contributions as a "theorist" transcended the domains of psychoanalysis and social psychology. In emphasizing this point, the purpose of his renowned book *Escape from Freedom* (1941) becomes evident.

Despite the common characterization of Fromm's writings as "simple" and straightforward, especially within Japanese academic discourse,[2] accurately discerning his thought is a challenging endeavor. This may be attributed to the fact that these writings are, in the truest sense of the word, highly interdisciplinary and not easily pigeonholed. For instance, Rainer Funk, a distinguished direct student of Fromm's, and others discern in Fromm's theory a "unique synthesis of Freudian, Marxist, sociological and Jewish radical intellectual traditions," thereby elucidating his extensive international readership, particularly with regard to *Escape from Freedom*.[3] However, as will be demonstrated subsequently, this "multidisciplinarity," as in the "unique synthesis," is both the essence of Fromm's theory and the primary rationale for the protracted academic oversight of his oeuvre. In summary, extant scholarship has identified Fromm's theoretical strengths as his weaknesses. In this sense, Fromm exemplifies a scholar whose reputation is clearly at odds with his contributions.

Nevertheless, Fromm's theory, especially within social theory, has garnered increasing appreciation in recent years for its interdisciplinary nature.[4] At the Third International Erich Fromm Research Congress in Berlin in 2018, Fromm's "social-psychoanalytic approach"[5] was met with significant acclaim, particularly following the reaffirmation of the objective of his theory to "bring… psychoanalysis and sociology together."[6] However, a significant

DOI: 10.4324/9781003600398-1

portion of the discourse did not constitute a continuation of Fromm's critical theory in its strict sense. The majority of these scholars were primarily concerned with the interpretation, analysis, and (clinical) application of Fromm's theory. It appeared that they did not have as their ultimate goal the development of his theory and the transformation of society through it (in the sense of the "improvement" of contemporary society).[7] However, it is precisely in this recognition that we may find in Fromm studies an opportunity for self-reflection and a potential solution to this problem.

In exploring the fundamental tenets of Fromm's theory from the aforementioned perspective, this book delves into the potential applications of his critical theory, while concurrently establishing a foundation for its theoretical and practical utility within the context of contemporary politics. The book's objective is twofold: first, to provide a comprehensive reconstruction of the critical theory foundations of Fromm's psychoanalysis, and second, to consider its "theory" implications.[8] To this end, the political theory indications of Fromm's theory are explored, particularly through a careful description of the process by which his early theory of analytical social psychology and his theory of narcissism were generated. This exploration portrays Fromm as a critical theorist who sought to explore the nature of democracy. He grappled with a pathological political form of fascism that emerged in early twentieth-century Central Europe. Fromm also sought to overcome this social pathology as a spiritual problem associated with "human nature."[9] In this regard, as we will see later, the "dialectic of narcissism" in Fromm's social theory, i.e., the psychoanalytical understanding of democracy in its dialectical relation to fascism, is central to his theory.[10]

In this introduction, I will first provide an overview of the current position of Fromm's theory and a brief look at the birth of Fromm as a critical theorist. In the following discussion, I will delineate three salient aspects of Fromm's theorizing that are pertinent to this book: a "theorist of narcissism," a "theorist of fascism," and a "theorist of democracy." The subsequent discussion will address the structural and organizational framework of the book.

## The Current Position of Fromm's Theory

As previously stated, Fromm is a personality whose work has historically received insufficient recognition within academic circles. Fromm is frequently designated a "forgotten intellectual,"[11] a clear indication that, despite his substantial contributions, he was consigned to a marginal role as a critical theorist and a Neo-Freudian. In particular, the focus on his former role has been overshadowed by the prominence of Horkheimer, Adorno, Habermas, and other related figures who were part of the Frankfurt School.

The apparent disregard for Fromm's contributions is further evidenced by the following observations. None of his theories has ever been given serious consideration by the mainstream of psychiatry and psychoanalysis.[12] This assertion is especially salient in the context of his theory of narcissism.[13] Yet this does not imply that Fromm's psychoanalytic theory is of substandard quality or unworthy of academic discourse. The predominant rationale for this phenomenon is the perception that his theory is unwieldy, particularly for disciplines that underwent increased compartmentalization during the twentieth century. This "unwieldiness" signifies that his theory does not conform readily to the subdivided disciplines. In the social context, Fromm's theory underscores the deleterious impact of the "marketplace mentality" on society and human existence.[14] However, this line of thinking is eschewed as a matter of principle, particularly in the advanced, market-based industrialized countries since the twentieth century. Ironically, in his early theoretical work, Fromm's dialectical and interdisciplinary theoretical endeavor of "analytic social psychology" ended up being neglected due to the fragmentation of academic fields, and he saw that mentality most manifested in the United States, the country to which he had emigrated. In this sense, Fromm was literally "confronted by estrangement and alienation everywhere."[15]

However, especially in the twenty-first century, there has been a reevaluation of Fromm's thought. As previously indicated, this phenomenon has been particularly evident in the field of social theory. While many of these reappraisals are certainly more revealing of the overall picture of Fromm's social theory than of individual themes, their common consciousness is undoubtedly that of Fromm as a critical theorist and a "disciple of Marx."[16] These aspects of Fromm's scholarly scheme are crucial to the very raison d'être of his social theory and are central to the theme of this book. The concept of "critique" is derived from these principles, thereby serving as the foundation for Fromm's social theory.[17]

However, it is the manner in which Fromm employs psychoanalysis that is more indicative of his critical theory. Of particular importance in this regard is his idiosyncratic characterological typology.[18] Fromm's theory of narcissism is a paradigmatic exemplar of this approach, serving a noteworthy archetype. The crux of his "critical" activities revolves around this characterological typology, but the most notable aspect of his oeuvre lies in the sociopsychological methodology that underlies his concepts of "individual character" and "social character."[19] This approach enables Fromm to identify and analyze social pathologies.

Despite the preeminence of Fromm's theory of "social character" in his theoretical scheme,[20] his theory of narcissism has gradually garnered increased attention. This is an additional long-ignored theory; nevertheless, it is indisputable that the rise of ethnonationalism and racial chauvinism in the political sphere of developed countries in recent years has begun to bring it into the limelight.[21] This finding lends credence to the notion that narcissism serves as a sociopsychological underpinning for various political movements, potentially contributing to the rise of populist politics. The observation underscores the relevance of Fromm's theory of narcissism, particularly in light of these findings. Consequently, the significance of his role as a critical theorist becomes evident in two distinct aspects: the recognition of the capacity of Fromm's critical theory to function as a social critique within the context of the present-day political landscape, and the potential of his theory of narcissism to contribute to critical theory.[22] For this reason, this book devotes particular attention to the possibility of a "Frommian critical social theory of narcissism."[23]

## A Theorist of Narcissism

Fromm is regarded as a "theorist of narcissism,"[24] primarily due to his self-identification as a "student of Freud"[25]—the concept of narcissism, which emerged predominantly from Freud's contributions, has been a central focus in Fromm's theoretical framework.[26] Narcissism is a quintessentially Freudian concept in this sense. Fromm's theory of narcissism, though, extends beyond the scope of Freud's in significant ways, especially with regard to its quantitative aspects. This is due to the fact that Fromm's theory is predicated on the interplay between social and individual levels. The term "social psychoanalyst" serves as a prime example of this phenomenon.[27]

The distinctive characteristic of Fromm's theory of narcissism is first and foremost its primary classification as a "characterological theory."[28] In essence, the concept of narcissism emerges in Fromm's theory as one of the distinct character types. According to the psychoanalyst Marco Bacciagaluppi, Fromm's theory of narcissism is characterized by three semantic pluralities: theoretical, sociopathological, and clinical.[29] The present book focuses on the second level, the sociopathological level, where Fromm's theory of narcissism is linked to another characterological theory, his unique concepts of "marketing orientation" and "having mode."[30] This phenomenon draws particular attention to the sociopathological function of the capitalist market society.

A distinguishing feature of Fromm's theory of narcissism at the sociopathological level is its profound association with the philosophical concept of "alienation," which emerged in nineteenth-century German philosophy.[31] This concept is a theory derived from Hegel and developed in particular by Marx.[32] Alienation is a sociopathological phenomenon that describes a social condition in which capital emerges as the subject of man, as man gradually loses his subjectivity with the development of capitalism.[33] Consequently, human beings are regarded as a commodity, and their role is limited to the production of surplus value in the form of labor power.[34] In Fromm's theoretical framework, this social pathology of alienation assumes the semantic role of the "marketing orientation," which is the character structure of market society—that is to say, the marketing orientation fulfills an economic function that is an integral component of the social function of alienation. Its function is defined as "I am as you desire me."[35] Moreover, the "having mode" previously referenced contributes to the phenomenon of alienation. This is rooted in the pursuit of material prosperity, as evidenced by the commitment to accumulate substantial material wealth: "put[ting] a lot of energies into having private property and thereby trying to satisfy oneself" (devoting the whole body to increasing possessions).[36] Of particular significance is the notion that narcissism, in its social manifestation, constitutes a psychological framework that enables an individual to "exist in a way that is preferred by others" within the economic sphere, and to "pour one's whole being into increasing one's possessions" within the subsistence realm. Fromm's theory posits that narcissism functions as a transference aimed at fulfilling the instinctual needs of a market economic society. In the context of an automotive metaphor, society can be conceptualized as the vehicle, while the market economy can be regarded as the engine that propels it. In this case, the marketing orientation and the having mode function as accelerators, and the personality structure of narcissism serves as the gear that makes this function possible. In this context, the individual operating the steering apparatus is designated as the driver, who is in control of the vehicle, though he or she is in a very passive position.

The above is a synopsis of Fromm's theory of narcissism, which is inherently intertwined with his social theory. However, as previously mentioned, Fromm's theory of narcissism has only recently come into vogue and has yet to be thoroughly explored from a theoretical perspective.[37] It affords considerable scope for delineation, and its prospective trajectory is contingent upon our collective discernment.

## A Theorist of Fascism

Fromm's theoretical perspective on fascism is deeply intertwined with the "interdisciplinary materialism" project at the Frankfurt Institute for Social Research, which was initiated in the early 1930s. Of particular importance in this discussion is the Institute's *Studien über Autorität und Familie* (1936).[38] Fromm's task was to detect "the father's role in the German middle-class bourgeois family."[39] This period marked the ascent of the Nazi Party to power in Germany. Concurrently, critical theorists, who had previously identified the fundamental issues within Nazi politics during the transfer of their research center to the United States, initiated an exploration of the socio-psychological underpinnings of these political problems. This exploration was undertaken from the distinctive vantage point of "authoritarianism."[40] Fromm was assigned to oversee a pivotal component of the project: the socio-psychological aspect.[41] According to Fromm, authoritarianism, which allegedly originated in the Western patriarchal family system, was linked to that at the social level through its manifestation at the family level. From Fromm's perspective, the social function of the family is the source of authoritarianism, specifically within the family unit.[42]

According to Fromm, the newly emergent middle class—consisting of twentieth-century workers who had come to represent a disintegrating nineteenth-century class society—sought support primarily from the Nazis because they could no longer bear the weight of their own isolated social condition, which had been caused by the rise of mass society. It has been posited that these individuals possessed authoritarian personality structures and engaged in unconsciously initiated sadomasochistic relationships, which paradoxically contributed to their success in transforming society. In essence, the concept of "authoritarian personality" served as an articulation of their form of social existence and a catalyst for the ascendance of the Nazi movement.[43] This notion functions as the overarching theme of Fromm's magnum opus, *Escape from Freedom*.

What has come to the fore in recent years, however, is the hidden presence in Fromm's theory of the character structure of narcissism underlying authoritarian politics, including fascism.[44] In the context of research on Fromm's theory of fascism, the concept of narcissism was infrequently addressed, with analysis instead focusing exclusively on authoritarianism, sadomasochism, and necrophilia (the love of death). However, it is crucial to acknowledge the significant influence of Fromm's psychoanalytic theory of narcissism on the understanding of fascist politics.[45] This theory, in its endeavor to comprehend narcissism through the lens of "human nature," offers a profound insight into the complex dynamics of fascist ideologies. In this sense, as previously mentioned, it is conceivable that Fromm's theory of narcissism is pertinent in the context of the recent rise of ethnonationalism and ethnic or racial chauvinism. From a methodological perspective, this could present an opportunity to surpass the limitations of conventional methods of fascist analysis. In the event that this is the case, *Escape from Freedom* can be reread from the perspective of traditional psychoanalysis. In this context, the potential for a "critical social theory of narcissism" emerges.

## A Theorist of Democracy

It is evident that Fromm's conceptualization of democracy, as outlined in *Escape from Freedom*, has significantly influenced his theoretical perspective. The book can be considered, in the strictest sense, his inaugural work of political theory. Although Fromm's conception of democracy is evident in the book, his later works, such as *Revolution of Hope* (1968) and *To Have or To Be?* (1976), are considered to be normative in terms of political theory. Thus, his subsequent years marked his emergence as a prominent political theorist.[46] This is not to imply, however, that Fromm had not evolved into a political theorist by the time *Escape from Freedom* was published. As would be anticipated, the efforts of Fromm to explore the meaning and possibilities of democracy are evident in this 1941 work, following his immigration to the United States in 1934. In essence, his inquiry into the concept of "freedom" within the paradigm of "individuality" represented an effort to discern the validity of democratic principles. This assertion underscores the significance of Fromm's contributions as a "theorist of democracy."

So what exactly was Fromm's take on American democracy? The subjugation of liberal democracy by the market mechanisms and the tenets of American democracy—the contradictions and limitations of liberal democracy—has been posited as a contributing factor to this phenomenon. The prevailing societal paradigm is characterized by a pervasive influence of the "market," encompassing the exchange of goods and services, as well as the concomitant values and behaviors that are inextricably linked to the underpinning character structures of a marketing orientation and a pervasive narcissistic culture. This experience prompted Fromm to adopt a position of total opposition to the market economy. Fromm's final sociotheoretical work, *To Have or To Be?*, is a clear expression of this position, which he maintained throughout his life.

It is therefore necessary to determine whether the various considerations previously enumerated can be utilized to ascertain the contemporary position of Fromm within the contemporary world. At this juncture, the objective of this discourse is to deliberate on three implications of Fromm's theory, particularly from the vantage point of social and political theory:

(1) The potential for a contemporary political analysis to employ Fromm's theory;[47]
(2) The normative theoretical potential of the theory;[48]
(3) The capacity to reevaluate the methodology of political theory through the lens of Fromm's sociopsychological methodology.[49]

It is noteworthy that all three perspectives have a direct bearing on the discipline of political theory.[50] In this sense, the focus on Fromm leads us to explore not only the possibility of developing philosophy, psychoanalysis, sociology, and social theory, which his theoretical scheme primarily encompasses, but also of developing political theory and its related fields of normative theory. Therefore, the significance of interpreting Fromm as a political theorist is contingent upon the analysis of contemporary politics and the updating of normative theory and methodology. From this perspective, significant opportunities for academic research on Fromm persist in the contemporary era. The extent to which we can benefit from this scholarship is dependent upon our recognition of these facts, our critical examination of his ideas, and our ability to contextualize and modernize them.

### Overview of Chapters

Chapter 1 offers bibliographical notes regarding Fromm's contributions. Firstly, the text provides a comprehensive overview of his sociopsychological contributions, particularly his seminal work, "The Method and Function of an Analytic Social Psychology" (1932), which was part of the early Frankfurt School project. Secondly, the chapter analyzes Fromm's seminal work, *Escape from Freedom*, elucidating its ascension to the status of his magnum opus and its reception beyond the confines of academia. Thirdly, it examines Fromm's later work, *To Have or To Be?*, focusing on the semantics of fascism depicted in the work. Ultimately, the objective of this chapter is to ascertain the meaning and significance of Fromm's writings.

Chapter 2 aims to shed light on Fromm's major theoretical contribution to the realm of political theory. The chapter commences with the presentation of his psychoanalytic theory as "sociological psychoanalysis."[51] The argument is posited that this phenomenon can be attributed to Fromm's distinctive sociological and psychoanalytic approach, which draws upon the theoretical contributions of Freud, Marx, and Weber. This approach was initially proposed by Fromm in 1932, and subsequently refined and expanded upon in his subsequent works. Secondly, the chapter expounds upon Fromm's conceptualization of authoritarianism, which is predicated on the aforementioned approach. It delves into the Institute for Social Research's *Studien über Autorität und Familie* (1936) and his seminal work *Escape from Freedom* (1941). Thirdly, the chapter examines Fromm's theory of alienation, a Marxist concept. This finding indicates a relationship between the theory and his other theories of "marketing orientation" and "having mode," which are understood characterologically.[52] Fourthly, it explores Fromm's socio-psychoanalytical conception of narcissism. Lastly, the chapter delineates Fromm's conceptualization of fascism, thereby underscoring its theoretical pertinence—the last section elucidates the contemporary implications of fascism in relation to Fromm's theory of authoritarianism. A comprehensive review of the extant literature reveals a high degree of pertinence of Fromm's theory to the contemporary political landscape, particularly with regard to the current resurgence of fascist political ideologies.

Chapter 3 examines the reception of Fromm's theory within the discipline of political theory, exploring the extent to which his contributions have been acknowledged. Firstly, the examination draws attention to research on authoritarianism, a concept/phenomenon that has been analyzed by a variety of disciplines, including political theory, social theory, philosophy, and many of the empirical social sciences. Secondly, an exploration of Fromm's concept of fascism is conducted within the context of relevant research, primarily from empirical disciplines such as sociology and political science. Thirdly, the concept of alienation is discussed, and the manner in which Fromm's conception of alienation has been treated in Marxism is illustrated.

Chapter 4 demonstrates the contemporary relevance of Fromm's political theory for today in relation to the concept of postfascism, a twenty-first-century form of fascism characterized by authoritarianism, nationalist protectionism, and anti-globalization, focusing on two representative Western democracies, the United States and Germany.[53] Firstly, the chapter delineates some pivotal political implications of Fromm's theories of narcissism and authoritarianism. Secondly, it conceptualizes the Frommian authoritarian-bureaucratic orientation, utilizing his conceptions of authoritarianism and bureaucracy. Thirdly, it elucidates the manner in which Fromm's political theory is related to the concept of postfascism. Fourthly, the text sheds light on postfascist politics, identifying its signification and problems within the democratic, postfascist political climate from a Frommian perspective. This book concludes that Fromm's political theory maintains its pertinence in the contemporary political landscape, particularly in the current political context of postfascism.

## Notes

1 Joan Braune, *Erich Fromm's Revolutionary Hope: Prophetic Messianism as a Critical Theory of the Future* (Rotterdam: Sense Publishers, 2014); Joan Braune and Kieran Durkin (Eds), *Erich Fromm's Critical Theory: Hope, Humanism, and the Future* (London: Bloomsbury Academic, 2020); Kieran Durkin, *The Radical Humanism of Erich Fromm* (New York: Palgrave Macmillan, 2014); Takamichi Sakurai, "A Frommian Perspective on the Socio-Psychological Structure of Post-Fascism in Liberal Democracies," *Distinktion: Journal of Social Theory*, 21, no. 2 (2020): 178–94.
2 Takayoshi Kitagawa and Takashi Miyajima (Eds), *Nijusseiki shakaigaku riron no tanjō* [The Birth of Twenty-Century Sociological Theory] (Tokyo: Yūshindō, 1996), 82.
3 Rainer Funk and Neil McLaughlin, "Introduction," in Funk and McLaughlin (Eds), *Towards a Human Science: The Relevance of Erich Fromm for Today* (Gießen: Psychosozial-Verlag, 2015), 15.
4 Braune, *Erich Fromm's Revolutionary Hope*; Braune and Durkin (Eds), *Erich Fromm's Critical Theory*; Durkin, *The Radical Humanism of Erich Fromm*; Michael Maccoby and Neil McLaughlin, "Sociopsychoanalysis and Radical Humanism: A Fromm-Bourdieu Synthesis," *Fromm Forum* (English edn.), 23 (2019): 45–57; Takamichi Sakurai, "The Authoritarian Orientation in Liberal Democracies: Labor Market and Workplace Authoritarianism," *Constellations* 32, no. 1 (2025): 59–68; Charles Thorpe, *Necroculture* (New York: Palgrave Macmillan, 2016).
5 Rainer Funk and Thomas Kühn, "Introduction," *Fromm Forum* (English edn.), 23 (2019): 5–8, at 6.
6 Rainer Funk, "Erich Fromm: Bringing Psychoanalysis and Sociology Together," *Fromm Forum* (English edn.), 23 (2019): 9–23; cf. Funk and Kühn, "Introduction."
7 It is evident that the early Frankfurt School's "critique" places significant emphasis on this notion of "transformation." (Max Horkheimer, "Traditional and Critical Theory," in Max Horkheimer, *Critical Theory: Selected Essays* (New York: Continuum, 2002 [1972]), 188–243; Max Horkheimer, "The Social Function of Philosophy," in M. Horkheimer (Ed.), *Critical Theory: Selected Essays* (New York: Continuum, 2002), 253–72.
8 In my opinion, the essence of "theory" lies first and foremost in provoking others. This is particularly evident in the negative reaction of an individual who might express bewilderment at the subject matter, such as by asking, "What on earth are you talking about?" The underlying reason for this phenomenon is that a theory that fails to surprise people and elicit a genuinely negative reaction cannot be expected to have any meaningful content as a "theory." Therefore, a theory that is effective in the sense of predicting some form of "change" generally possesses elements that irritate people. I believe that a seminal aspect of "critical theory," one that is of profound epistemological significance, resides precisely in this juncture.
9 Takamichi Sakurai, *Political Theories of Narcissism: Towards Self-Reflections on Knowledge and Politics from the Psychoanalytic Perspectives of Erich Fromm and Fujita Shōzō* (Zurich: LIT Verlag, 2018), ch. 6, Sect. 6.4.
10 Sakurai, *Political Theories of Narcissism*, 176–93; Takamichi Sakurai, "The Socio-Psychological Base of Contemporary Fascism in the World of Liberal Democracy: The Theoretical Scope of Erich Fromm's Socio-Pathological Theory of Alienation," *Fromm Forum* (English edn.), 22 (2018): 143–55, at 150–52.

11 Neil McLaughlin, "How to Become a Forgotten Intellectual: Intellectual Movements and the Rise and Fall of Erich Fromm," *Sociological Forum*, 13 (1998): 215–46; Neil McLaughlin, "Who Killed off Fromm's Reputation in North America? Russell Jacoby's Social Amnesia and the Forgetting of a Public Intellectual," *Fromm Forum* (English edn.), 21 (2017): 7–21, at 12.
12 Sakurai, *Political Theories of Narcissism*, 148–9.
13 Sakurai, *Political Theories of Narcissism*, 148–9.
14 Ruth Lesser, "Erich Fromm and the Psychoanalysis of the Social Unconscious," *Fromm Forum* (English edn.), 6 (2002): 23–24, at 24.
15 József Koch, "Erich Fromm's Humanistic View of Man and Our Divided World," Paper for the International Erich Fromm Society's seminar on Character Structure and Society, Janus Pannonius University, Hungary, 24–26 August 1990 (retrieved from: http://opus4.kobv.de/opus4-Fromm/files/13699/Koch_J_1990c.pdf).
16 For example, Mary Rattray, "Erich Fromm: A Twentieth Century Prophet?" (M.Th. Thesis, University of Glasgow, 1995), 94, 272.
17 For "critique" in Fromm, see Erich Fromm, *Beyond the Chains of Illusion: My Encounter with Marx and Freud* (London: Abacus, 1962); for "critique" in the Frankfurt School, Horkheimer, "Traditional and Critical Theory"; Horkheimer, "The Social Function of Philosophy."
18 Erich Fromm, "Psychoanalytic Characterology and Its Application to the Understanding of Culture," in S. Stansfeld Sargent and Marian W. Smith (Eds), *Culture and Personality* (New York: Viking Fund, 1949), 1–12.
19 Fromm, *Beyond the Chains of Illusion*, ch. 8; Erich Fromm, "Über Methode und Aufgaben einer analytischen Sozialpsychologie. Bemerkungen über Psychoanalyse und historischen Materialismus," in Rainer Funk (Ed.), *Erich Fromm Gesamtausgabe, Band 1: Analytische Sozialpsychologie* (Stuttgart: Deutsche Verlags-Anstalt, 1980 [1932]), 37–57.
20 Uschi Essbach-Kreuzer, "Die Theorie des Sozialcharakters in den Arbeiten von Erich Fromm," in Adelbert Reif (Hg.), *Erich Fromm: Materialien zu seinem Werk* (Wien: Europa Verlag, 1978), 299–326; Rainer Funk, "Erich Fromm's Concept of Social Character and Its Relevance for Clinical Practice," in Mauricio Cortina and Michael Maccoby (Eds), *A Prophetic Analyst: Erich Fromm's Contribution to Psychoanalysis* (Northvale and London: Jason Aronson, 1996), 341–60; Alan Grey, "Society as Destiny: Fromm's Concept of Social Character," *Contemporary Psychoanalysis*, 28, no. 2 (1992): 344–63; Luis Jimenez, "Revisiting Fromm's Concept of Social Character and Social Change: An Example from De-Industrialized Working Class Communities in the UK," *Fromm Forum*, 23 (2019): 182–98; Michael Maccoby, "Toward a Science of Social Character," *International Forum of Psychoanalysis*, 11, no. 1 (2002): 33–44; Salvador Millán, "The Third World and the Social Character," in International Erich Fromm Society (Ed.), *Wissenschaft vom Menschen/Science of Man*, vol. 3 (Münster: LIT Verlag, 1992), 57–67; Dale H. Ortmeyer, "Clinical Relevance of Social Character and Social Unconscious," *International Forum of Psychoanalysis*, 11, no. 1 (2002): 4–9; Tatiana Panfilova, "Social Character and Social Unconscious: Erich Fromm's Discovery and the Problems of Today," in Rainer Funk and Neil McLaughlin (Eds), *Towards a Human Science: The Relevance of Erich Fromm for Today* (Gießen: Psychosozial-Verlag, 2015), 201–7.
21 For example, see Takeshi Deguchi, "Post-Truth Politics as a Pathology of Normalcy: Beyond Alienation and Narcissism in the Age of Globalization," *Fromm Forum*, 23 (2019): 161–68; Patrick Ehnis and Katrin Voigt, "Fromm's Contribution to the Analysis and Critique of the Ongoing Rise of Right-Wing Movements," *Fromm Forum*, 23 (2019): 138–52; Douglas Kellner, *American Nightmare: Donald Trump, Media Spectacle, and Authoritarian Populism* (Rotterdam: Sense Publishers, 2016); Douglas Kellner, "Donald Trump as Authoritarian Populist: A Frommian

Analysis," in Jeremiah Morelock (Ed.), *Critical Theory and Authoritarian Populism* (London: University of Westminster Press, 2018); Sakurai, "The Socio-Psychological Base of Contemporary Fascism in the World of Liberal Democracy"; Sakurai, "A Frommian Perspective on the Socio-Psychological Structure of Post-Fascism in Liberal Democracies"; Thorpe, *Necroculture.*

22 Deguchi, "Post-Truth Politics as a Pathology of Normalcy"; Kellner, "Donald Trump as Authoritarian Populist"; Sakurai, "The Socio-Psychological Structure of Post-Fascism in Liberal Democracies."

23 Deguchi, "Post-Truth Politics as a Pathology of Normalcy"; Sakurai, "The Socio-Psychological Structure of Post-Fascism in Liberal Democracies"; Sakurai, "The Authoritarian Orientation in Liberal Democracies."

24 Sakurai, *Political Theories of Narcissism*; Sakurai, "The Socio-Psychological Structure of Post-Fascism in Liberal Democracies."

25 Richard I. Evans, *Dialogue with Erich Fromm* (New York: Harper and Row, 1966), 59.

26 Sigmund Freud, "On Narcissism: An Introduction," in James Strachey (Ed. and Trans.), *The Standard Edition of the Complete Psychological Works of Sigmund Freud*, vol. 14 (London: Hogarth Press, 2001 [1953]), 67–102; cf. Kenneth Levy, William D. Ellison, and Joseph S. Reynoso, "A Historical Review of Narcissism and Narcissistic Personality," in W. Keith Campbell and Joshua D. Miller (Eds), *The Handbook of Narcissism and Narcissistic Personality Disorder: Theoretical Approaches, Empirical Findings, and Treatments* (Hoboken, NJ: John Wiley & Sons, 2011), 3–13; Sakurai, *Political Theories of Narcissism*, Appendix 2.

27 Rainer Funk, *Das Leben selbst ist eine Kunst. Einführung in Leben und Werk von Erich Fromm*, Neuausgabe (Freiburg: Herder, 2018), 70; cf. Funk, "Erich Fromm."

28 Erich Fromm, *Man for Himself: An Inquiry into the Psychology of Ethics* (London: Routledge & Kegan Paul, 1997 [1947]); Erich Fromm, *The Art of Loving* (New York and Evanston: Harper & Row, 1962 [1956]); Erich Fromm, *The Heart of Man: Its Genius for Good and Evil* (New York: Harper & Row, 1964); cf. Marco Bacciagaluppi, "Fromm's Views on Narcissism and the Self," in John Fiscalini and Alan L. Grey (Eds), *Narcissism and the Interpersonal Self* (New York: Columbia University Press, 1993), 91–106; John Fiscalini, *Narcissism and Self-Disorder*, in Marylou Lionells, John Fiscalini, Carola Mann, and Donnel B. Stern (Eds), *Handbook of Interpersonal Psychoanalysis* (New York and London: Routledge, 2009), 333–74.

29 Bacciagaluppi, "Fromm's Views on Narcissism and the Self."

30 Fromm, *Man for Himself*; Erich Fromm, *To Have or To Be?* (New York: Continuum, 2011 [1976]); Sakurai, *Political Theories of Narcissism*, ch. 6, sect. 6.3.

31 Sakurai, *Political Theories of Narcissism*, 169–77; Sakurai, "The Socio-Psychological Base of Contemporary Fascism in the World of Liberal Democracy"; Sakurai, "The Authoritarian Orientation in Liberal Democracies."

32 Sean Sayers, *Marx and Alienation: Essays on Hegelian Themes* (Basingstoke and New York: Palgrave Macmillan, 2011); Richard Schacht, *The Future of Alienation* (Urbana and Chicago: University of Illinois Press, 1994).

33 Karl Marx, *Capital, vol. 1: A Critique of Political Economy*, Ben Fowkes (Trans.) (London: Penguin Classics, 1992 [1867]); Karl Marx, *Economic and Philosophical Manuscripts*, Thomas B. Bottomore (Trans.), in Erich Fromm (Ed.), *Marx's Concept of Man* (London: Bloomsbury Academic, 2013 [1844]).

34 Marx, *Capital, vol. 1: A Critique of Political Economy*; Marx, *Economic and Philosophical Manuscripts*.

35 Fromm, *Man for Himself*, 72–73.

36 Sakurai, "The Authoritarian Orientation in Liberal Democracies," 61.

37 It is important to acknowledge that Fromm's theory of narcissism persists in being overlooked by the prevailing psychoanalytic discourse.

38 Institut für Sozialforschung (Ed.), *Studien über Autorität und Familie* (Paris: Alcan, 1936); Erich Fromm, "Sozialpsychologischer Teil," in Institut für Sozialforschung (Ed.), *Studien über Autorität und Familie*; Erich Fromm et al., "Zweite Abteilung. Erhebungen," in Institut für Sozialforschung (Ed.), *Studien über Autorität und Familie*.
39 Fromm, "Sozialpsychologischer Teil"; Fromm et al., "Zweite Abteilung."
40 Institut für Sozialforschung (Ed.), *Studien über Autorität und Familie*.
41 For example, see Annette Thomson, *Erich Fromm: Shaper of the Human Condition* (London: Palgrave Macmillan, 2009), 10.
42 Fromm, "Sozialpsychologischer Teil."
43 Fromm, *Escape from Freedom*.
44 Sakurai, *Political Theories of Narcissism*, ch. 6, sect. 6.4; Sakurai, "The Socio-Psychological Base of Contemporary Fascism in the World of Liberal Democracy"; Sakurai, "The Authoritarian Orientation in Liberal Democracies."
45 It is evident that narcissism plays a pivotal role in Fromm's theory of fascism; however, this has seldom been acknowledged. This is likely attributable to the fact that Fromm does not overtly employ the term "narcissism" in his theoretical framework concerning fascism.
46 It is important to note that, irrespective of one's specialization in the academic discipline of "political theory," all human beings possess the potential to engage in the practice of political theory—in this sense, it is not obligatory to be a "political theorist." This assertion is applicable to Fromm's contributions as well. The rationale for emphasizing this point is twofold. Firstly, within the prevailing context of profound specialization in academic domains, the designation "...ologist" or "...ist" is predominantly determined by the specific discipline of expertise. Secondly, within a democratic system, citizens are expected to partake in a range of political activities and exercises of civic duty.
47 For example, see Kellner, *American Nightmare: Donald Trump, Media Spectacle, and Authoritarian Populism*; Kellner, "Donald Trump as Authoritarian Populist"; Sakurai, *Political Theories of Narcissism*, "The Authoritarian Orientation in Liberal Democracies."
48 For example, see Durkin, *The Radical Humanism of Erich Fromm*; Michael J. Thompson, "Normative Humanism and Redemptive Critique: Knowledge and Judgment in Erich Fromm's Social Theory," in Seyed Javad Miri, Robert Lake, and Tricia M. Kress (Eds), *Reclaiming the Sane Society: Essays on Erich Fromm's Thought* (Rotterdam: Sense Publishers, 2014), 37–58; Lawrence Wilde, *Erich Fromm and the Quest for Solidarity* (Houndmills, Basingstoke, Hampshire: Palgrave Macmillan, 2004).
49 Sakurai, *Political Theories of Narcissism*.
50 In my experience, it is challenging to identify political theorists who are actively involved in the Fromm circle in the literal sense. It is noteworthy that the only political theorists who can be said to be engaged in the aforementioned circle are Lawrence Wilde and Michael J. Thompson. The biases stemming from the specialized fields of the scholars involved with this community—psychoanalysis, psychiatry, psychology, sociology, and philosophy—still exert influence on its formation and activities.
51 Sakurai, *Political Theories of Narcissism*, 217; cf. Grey, "Society as Destiny."
52 Fromm, *Man for Himself*; *To Have or to Be* (1976).
53 Sakurai, "A Frommian Perspective on the Socio-Psychological Structure of Post-Fascism in Liberal Democracies"; Takamichi Sakurai, "The Socio-Theoretical Relevance of Erich Fromm's Psychoanalytic Conception of Narcissism: Towards a Frommian Critical Social Theory of Narcissism," *Theoria: A Journal of Social and Political Theory*, 68, no. 166 (2021): 1–30; Takamichi Sakurai, "Aspirational Fascism versus Postfascism: A Conceptual History of a Far-Right Politics," *History of European Ideas*, 48, no. 5 (2022): 650–60; Enzo Traverso, *The New Faces of Fascism* (London: Verso, 2019).

# 1 A Comprehensive Overview of Fromm's Primary Works

## The Birth of Erich Fromm as a Critical Theorist

### *The Early Project of the Frankfurt School*

Fromm was born on March 23, 1900, in the German Empire of Wilhelm II. The city of Frankfurt, where he was born and raised, had lost its independent function as a free city to the Prussian invasion and was in the process of annexing surrounding cities and towns to become an emblematic cosmopolitan city of Western Europe. Fromm's upbringing was marked by the privilege of being the eldest son of a Jewish wine merchant in an opulent neighborhood of Westend. Perhaps his character is best illustrated by his own question: "What is it that makes people think, feel, and act so irrationally?"[1] Fromm must have had an active personality that allowed him to question and express himself in any way he chose, as Rainer Funk has often pointed out. He may have been influenced by the strict upbringing of his father and the liberal and humanistic views of Rabinkov, his tutor. This positive character is evident in his dissertation, "Jewish Law: Toward a Sociology of the Diaspora," which Fromm submitted to the University of Heidelberg in 1922.[2]

Meanwhile, Germany entered World War I as a major ally in 1914, only to surrender to the Allies in 1918. Shortly before the end of World War I, the German Revolution was already in full swing, and by 1919, Germany would be in transition to the Weimar Republic. However, the Weimar Republic, which had not only allowed the military and monopoly capital to remain in Germany, but had also been forced to establish itself with a large number of discontented elements, created the image of a huge scapegoat in society, especially as the number of people who blamed communism and Jewish elements for the failure of the First World War grew day by day. Hitler, who was of Austrian origin, famously entered Weimar Germany through Bavaria and further strengthened the ideological movement of national chauvinism. He became a German citizen in 1932 and was officially recognized as President of Germany by the parliament in 1933.

Obviously, someone like Fromm would be at a particular disadvantage under such social conditions. Although Fromm was conducting research at the Institute for Social Research in Frankfurt at the time, it did not take him long to decide that his best option was to use his social roots to flee the

DOI: 10.4324/9781003600398-2

country. In 1934, he and members of the Institute fled to the United States via Geneva. The reason that Fromm remained abnormally attached to Freud even after he resumed his research activities in the United States was not only because he thought that Freud's instinct theory would enrich Marx's dialectical critique, but rather because he thought that it would offer a crucial insight into the comprehension of Nazism. The early Frankfurt School was a critical source of information in this sense. It is imperative to know that the project of "interdisciplinary materialism" of the early Frankfurt School undoubtedly had a serious historical background related to the origins of its members, as outlined above, and that the meaning of "critique" was condensed in it.[3] For Fromm, the sense of "critique," as he would later articulate it, is the realization of the development of democracy in "a society in which the individual, his growth and happiness, is the aim and purpose of culture."[4] Fromm calls this the "victory of freedom."[5] But it is the Germans, especially after World War I, who destroyed it with their own hands, relying on a different meaning of "freedom" (negative freedom) than this meaning of "freedom" (positive freedom), Fromm asserts. The continuation of this important work of "critique" in this book is a Frommian critical social theory of narcissism.

### *Analytic Social Psychology*

Fromm's "analytic social psychology" occupies a pivotal position in the early corpus of his works. It is evident that the development of analytic social psychology in Fromm constitutes a seminal contribution to his subsequent scholarly endeavors. His conceptualization of narcissism, as articulated in this book, draws considerable influence from the tenets of analytic social psychology. However, a comprehensive examination of Fromm's analytic social psychology has been conspicuously absent from extant scholarship. As elaborated below, while there has been a modicum of attention devoted to this seminal work of early Fromm, it must be acknowledged that few other works have encapsulated its essence with the same precision. This observation stands as a testament to the current state of Fromm's analytic social psychology.

Conversely, a substantial body of research has emerged on Fromm's concept of "social character." This phenomenon can be attributed to the fact that Fromm was the first to utilize and elucidate the concept in his seminal work, *Escape from Freedom*. Hence, it is not surprising that individuals who read Fromm and are interested in his thought would want to know about "social character." However, a comprehensive understanding of "social character" necessitates a review of his extant writings preceding *Escape from Freedom*. This is due to the fact that the establishment of his method of analytic social psychology, which served as the foundation for early Fromm's methodology, had already been accomplished by the time he wrote the book *Escape from Freedom*. This methodology was employed to elucidate the significance of Fromm's array of sociopsychological concepts, including social character. This seminal work was undertaken in his "Methods and Functions of Analytical Social Psychology" (1932) (henceforth "ASP"). Nevertheless,the work has received scant attention from Fromm scholars, particularly in the context of social character. Instead, the majority of these scholars have directed their attention to the subsequent works of Fromm, particularly *Escape from Freedom.*

Fromm's book *Escape from Freedom* is notable for its omission of any theoretical consideration of the concept of social character.[6] This omission suggests that Fromm effectively applied the concept of social character in the book. Namely, in his subsequent research endeavors, Fromm's primary focus transitioned from addressing "methodological concerns" in social psychology to exploring societal dynamics. Following the completion of his methodological examination of social character, Fromm employed the concept with renewed confidence in *Escape from Freedom.* As will be demonstrated subsequently, Fromm's presentation of the concept of "social need" in *Escape from Freedom* can be regarded as a dismissal of Freud's instinctive theory. A notable distinction emerges between "ASP" and *Escape from Freedom*, a point that is crucial to understanding the evolution of Fromm's conception of analytic social psychology. However, the central focus of this chapter lies elsewhere. Instead, the present chapter will focus on the theoretical implications of Fromm's concept of social character. The objective of this chapter is to identify the most salient theoretical tenets of analytic social psychology.

In view of the foregoing considerations, it becomes essential to elucidate the rationale behind Fromm's decision to base his research endeavors on "social psychology," a field that does not fall under the purview of either sociology or psychology. Indeed, this very question constitutes the primary concern of Fromm's methodological position in social psychology, his analytical social psychology. A notable observation is that his article "ASP" is subtitled "A Note on Psychoanalysis and Historical Materialism." This subtitle is pivotal in addressing the aforementioned inquiry. In essence, Fromm's objective in this seminal work is to establish a nexus between Freud and Marx, delving into the underlying reasons behind Marx's *appeal* to Freud. Fromm sought to demonstrate in the article that Marx's historical materialism required psychoanalysis to be fully explicated. It is noteworthy that, within the academic milieu of the early 1930s, this perspective was regarded as heretical, with the exception of those who could be classified as Western Marxists and a select few who influenced Fromm, such as Wilhelm Reich.

### *The Relevance and Problems of Fromm's Analytic Social Psychology*

It is imperative to elucidate the theoretical significance of analytic social psychology. A notable accomplishment of analytic social psychology is its contribution to the accessibility of psychoanalysis within the domain of the social sciences. This achievement stems from the ability of the methodological framework of analytic social psychology to overcome the profound and entrenched dialectical contradiction that existed between the methodological incompatibility of traditional sociology and traditional psychology. By addressing this challenge, analytic social psychology has facilitated the development of Fromm's original method, thereby fostering a more comprehensive and integrated understanding of psychoanalysis within the context of the social sciences.

Nevertheless, the dialectic of analytic social psychology has not yet undergone complete sublimation. This is attributable to an inherent problem in Fromm's conceptualization of "psychoanalytic social psychology." This field deviates from the conventional conception of "social psychology" due to its marked differences with the empirical social psychology that emerged particularly in the early twentieth century. Fromm's "psychoanalytic social psychology," which was formed at a considerable distance from the concept of "social psychology" that can be seen from the juxtaposition of "psychological social psychology" and "sociological social psychology," which existed until the 1960s, can almost never be lumped into the scope of "social psychology" seen in parallel with the rise of positivism and behaviorism.[7] Concurrently, this observation underscores the fact that Fromm's conception of social psychology has become inaccessible to the prevailing positivist social psychology (since the 1970s, psychological social psychology has predominated). Consequently, this shift has given rise to a notable degree of skepticism, particularly given the foundation of his "social psychology" in psychoanalysis. Secondly, the issue of Fromm's position of "sociological psychoanalysis," constructed by the methods of analytical social psychology, complicates matters further.[8] While this has undoubtedly facilitated a cross-fertilization between sociology and psychoanalysis, it has also created a significant impediment to the integration of psychoanalysis within the sociological framework. This issue is exemplified by the observation that most psychoanalytic theories do not engage the social.[9] In my estimation, this predicament is most aptly illustrated by the challenge of operationalizing Fromm's concept of "social character" from a psychoanalytic vantage point.

A thorough examination of the criticisms leveled at Fromm's approach in analytical social psychology reveals that the issues identified therein are not exhaustive. Firstly, the limitation of Fromm's employment of the term "psychology" is problematic. Secondly, the conceptual limitations and specificity of "individual psychology" and "social psychology" in Fromm's theoretical framework pose challenges in comprehending the entirety of his contributions. Fromm's exclusive identification of psychology with Freud's ego psychology, excluding alternative psychological systems, is problematic. In essence, when Fromm employs the term "psychology," he is referring exclusively to the framework of classical psychoanalysis, thereby delineating a highly constrained definition of psychology. Consequently, Fromm's employment of the term "psychology" is remarkably constrained. Addressing the second issue, it is crucial to note that Fromm's conceptualization of "individual psychology" and "social psychology" as mere paraphrases of Freudian ego psychology and modified ego psychology (sociological ego psychology in Fromm's terms) underscores the extreme limitations and specificity of his usage of these terms. This limitation is closely related to the first problem, especially in the sense that, in Fromm's thought, the term "psychology" is used only in that it is joined to Marx's theory of socioeconomic structure through Weber's individualistic sociology under the connotation of Freudian ego psychological psychoanalysis. For this reason, when examining Fromm's psychological concepts, it is vital to pay particular attention to their conceptual limitation and specificity.

Notwithstanding the aforementioned two issues, Fromm's analytical social psychology remains highly significant in the present day. The significance of his social psychology is demonstrated by its dialectical relationship to the aforementioned problems. The merits of analytical social psychology are contingent upon its limitations, and conversely, the limitations of analytical social psychology are contingent upon its merits. Fromm's theoretical contributions to social psychology, as articulated in his foundational methodology, entail the establishment of a distinct value system that integrates Freudian psychoanalysis and Marxian economic and social structure theory. This value system is distinctly separate from the paradigm of empirical science and serves as a foundational framework for psychoanalysis informed by sociological theory. The contemporary significance of this work lies in its potential to offer a reflective perspective on Fromm's social psychology within the context of positivist social psychology and to facilitate "self-reflection" based on the social aspects of his psychoanalysis.

### *Escape from Freedom* (1941)

Fromm's book *Escape from Freedom* is widely regarded as his magnum opus, and it has garnered a substantial international audience. It is noteworthy that the same book was published under the title *The Fear of Freedom* (1941), which was later translated into German as *Die Angst vor der Freiheit* (1952)—the latter English title appears to align more closely with Fromm's intended semantic meaning of the book.

It is broadly acknowledged that Fromm authored this book during his subsequent life in the United States, following his immigration from Germany. Fromm's capacity to relocate to another country in the early twentieth century indicates a significant degree of privilege. However, it is plausible to hypothesize that the transition for Fromm, a German national, to write in English, a foreign language, represented a significant challenge. Notably, *Escape from Freedom*, Fromm's inaugural book, was also his first written in English.

The book's foundational premise is the concept of authoritarianism, its operational mechanisms, and the conceptualization of a pathological politics. In this book, Fromm employs psychoanalysis to examine the dynamics of politics, elucidating the role of sadomasochism in authoritarian politics and, by extension, fascism. This approach constitutes a significant departure from prevailing thought at the time. Fromm's focus on Nazi politics and its mechanisms of operation is evident. It is noteworthy, however, that while critiquing the Nazi regime, Fromm's focus was on the American market society—this is an alternative interpretation of *Escape from Freedom*. From Fromm's perspective, the book was written from an American vantage point. Nonetheless, Fromm's primary objective in his work is arguably to meticulously analyze the sociopsychological underpinnings of the political transformation from the Weimar Republic to the Third Reich and the psychology of Nazism. In this endeavor, he seeks to illuminate the factors that led to Germany's descent into fascism and to propose a strategy for fortifying democracy. A close examination of the book's three fundamental themes—sadomasochism, authoritarianism, and freedom—is therefore warranted.

### *Sadomasochism*

Fromm's theoretical framework regarding sadomasochism is fundamentally predicated on the notion of symbiosis and incestuous bonds. A thorough elucidation of this conception was previously delineated in the Introduction. The subsequent discourse will therefore offer a synopsis of the salient points.

In *Escape from Freedom*, Fromm presents the argument that the authoritarian character structure, which serves as the foundational basis of fascist political ideologies, is characterized by the pathological manifestation of sadomasochistic symbiosis. From this perspective, within the context of this symbiotic human relationship, individuals develop a pathological dependence on each other, giving rise to a sadomasochistic desire that is primarily driven by feelings of unbearable loneliness. This phenomenon, marked by the intensification of social isolation and the rise of mass society, has emerged as a consequence of the atomization of individuals within contemporary society. Fromm asserts that this phenomenon constitutes the primary factor in a sociopathological occurrence, wherein individuals are compelled to establish a "secondary bond."[10] He proposes that this alternative to "primary bonds," which people have historically relied on for autonomy, functions as a catalyst for individuals to evade the psychological state of loneliness, irrespective of any loss of personal freedom. This phenomenon, he contends, fosters the formation of social bonds among individuals under mass social conditions.[11] As Fromm articulates, "his active solidarity with all men and his spontaneous activity, love and work…unite him again with the world, not by primary ties but as a free and independent individual."[12] In Fromm's social theory, the concept of an incestuous tie signifies a pathological phenomenon characterized by the consolidation of individuals within a cohesive structure. This tie functions as a manifestation of an authoritarian drive, encompassing both a sadistic component, characterized by the pursuit of control over subordinates, and a masochistic element, involving the transference of personal vulnerabilities to authority figures. This superiority is not merely a means of seizing power, but rather an inherent dependency between the individual and their raison d'être. As Fromm theorizes, individuals who manifest sadistic and masochistic inclinations frequently exhibit a propensity toward authoritarianism.

### *Authoritarianism*

In *Escape from Freedom*, Fromm's analysis of authoritarianism is constrained to its interpretation as sadomasochistic symbiosis, as mentioned above. However, this concept is subsequently associated with "necrophilia," particularly in his literary work, *The Anatomy of Human Destructiveness*, published in 1973. In this exposition, the central tenets of the aforementioned discourse will be distilled for the sake of brevity.

In this seminal text, Fromm advanced his theory of authoritarianism, delving more profoundly into the clinical and pathological dimensions of authoritarianism. A notable facet of the analysis involves the application of the concept of necrophilia to the discourse on fascism, a strategy that merits further examination. Fromm's perspective posits that necrophilia is the "love of the dead."[13] This concept is theorized to be classified into two distinct categories: the former category, termed "sexual necrophilia," defined as a "man's desire to have sexual intercourse or any other kind of sexual contact with a female corpse," while the latter, "nonsexual necrophilia," is characterized as the "desire to handle, to be near to, and to gaze at corpses, and particularly the desire to disremember them."[14] Fromm's emphasis on this concept of necrophilia is indicative of his endeavor to establish a connection between the pathological concept and his characterological theory. The "necrophilous character" is characterized as a "passionate attraction to all that is dead, decayed, putrid, sickly."[15] This definition is attributed to Hans von Hentig, a renowned German criminal psychologist.

Fromm's analysis of Hitler's character accentuates his proclivity for necrophilia. He is portrayed as a paradigmatic necrophilous individual, driven by the compulsion to "transform a man into a corpse."[16] Accordingly, human beings characterized by a necrophilous orientation, as posited by Fromm in his analysis of Adolf Hitler, are driven to destroy the very fabric of existence through the implementation of force. As Fromm asserts, "[w]hat has been, i.e., what is dead, rules his life: institutions, laws, property, traditions, and possessions."[17] Consequently, as Fromm contends, "*things rule man; having rules being; the dead rule the living.*"[18] In this context, tangible entities such as things and human beings are conspicuously absent, and instead, abstract entities are utilized merely as instruments of force. From these vantage points, necrophilia is characterized particularly by destruction. A deleterious aspect of the character is associated with "sadism," and, by extension, with authoritarianism.[19] Fromm's theoretical contributions to the study of fascism merit particular attention, as he advanced a pathological clinical concept for the political analysis of fascism.

### *Two Distinct Categories of Freedoms*

In Fromm's social and political theory, the concept of freedom is classified into two distinct categories: "freedom from" represents negative freedom, while "freedom to" represents positive freedom. The latter is deemed salient in the context of democracy. The former signifies the act of liberating oneself from constraints, that is to say, the act of extricating oneself from the conditions that confine an individual, such as incarceration. The latter signifies the endeavor to proactively partake in the political process with the objective of promoting societal well-being. Fromm places significant emphasis on the latter aspect, underscoring the manner in which human beings engage with "productive work."[20] In the context of politics, this dynamic establishes a substantial foundation for democratic systems.

In order to ascertain the substance of these two freedoms, it is necessary to utilize Fromm's methodological stance on dialectical analysis, as it is instrumental in this endeavor. Fromm's consistent adoption of a dialectical perspective throughout his oeuvre is a reasonable postulation. The following sentence exemplifies his dialectical method.

> [m]an, the more he gains freedom in the sense of emerging from the original oneness with man and nature and the more he becomes an "individual," has no choice but to unite himself with the world in the spontaneity of love and productive work or else to seek a kind of security by such ties with the world as destroy his freedom and the integrity of his individual self.[21]

Notably, the concept articulated by *Escape from Freedom* concerning the dialectical evolution of politics has received minimal scholarly attention.[22] This has led to a prevalent misapprehension regarding the nature of *Escape from Freedom*. The prevailing interpretation of the text is that it offers a rudimentary critique of fascism (Nazism).[23] This misapprehension stems from an oversight in recognizing that Fromm's academic undertakings are, in essence, executed through the utilization of the dialectical method. This philosophical device is crucially important because it reveals that, in some ways, democracy and fascism have functional similarities. A foundational element of Fromm's theoretical framework is the pervasive presence of dialectic, a concept that serves as a pivotal nexus between his theory and critical theory.[24]

While Fromm's ostensible objective in the book is to propose a solution to Nazism, his true intention is much more profound. The crux of the matter pertains to the fundamental essence of human existence. In the specific context of contemporary society, Fromm proposes the hypothesis that humans have become objects of the capitalist system. In this regard, it is essential to acknowledge the fundamental existential implications of the contemporary phenomenon of alienation. The influence of this phenomenon engenders in the individual the perception that one is a means of fulfilling one's own needs to satisfy them; consequently, one becomes a means of maintaining one's own existence. In essence, the fundamental nature of human existence has undergone a profound reinterpretation, reducing individuals to mere components of the "labor power" apparatus, which is deemed indispensable for generating surplus value. This process is marked by a paradoxical phenomenon that not only diminishes human autonomy but is also fundamental to the system's operation.

The human condition is defined by the manner in which individuals address the *existential contradictions* that are distinctive to their experience. In this regard, Fromm's perspective on the nexus between "human existence" and "freedom" merits attention.

> Human existence begins when the lack of fixation of action by instincts exceeds a certain point; when the adaptation to nature loses its coercive character; when the way to act is no longer fixed by hereditarily given mechanisms. In other words, *human existence and freedom are from the beginning inseparable*.[25]

Fromm's perspective on human existence serves as a critical component of my investigation into the political implications of "freedom" within his theoretical framework. Fromm employs a narrative strategy to elucidate the process by which human beings form their own cultural identities by utilizing the creation narrative as recounted in the *Book of Genesis* (The Creation Story):

> The myth identifies the beginning of human history with an act of choice, but it puts all emphasis on the sinfulness of this first act of *freedom* and the suffering resulting from it. Man and woman live in the Garden of Eden in complete harmony with each other and with nature. There is peace and no necessity to work; there is no choice, no *freedom*, no thinking either. Man is forbidden to eat from the tree of knowledge of good and evil. He acts against God's command, he breaks through the state of harmony with nature of which he is a part without transcending it. From the standpoint of the Church which represented authority, this is essentially sin. From the standpoint of man, however, this is the beginning of human *freedom*. Acting against God's orders means freeing himself from coercion, emerging from the unconscious existence of prehumen life to the level of man. Acting against the command of authority, committing a sin, is in its positive human aspect the first act of *freedom*, that is, the first human act. In the myth the sin in its formal aspect is the acting against God's command; in its material aspect it is the eating of the tree of knowledge. The act of disobedience as an act of *freedom* is the beginning of reason. The myth speaks of other consequences of the first act of *freedom*. The original harmony between man and nature is broken. God proclaims war between man

> and woman, and war between nature and man. Man has become separate from nature, he has taken the first step toward becoming human by becoming an "individual." He has committed the first act of *freedom*. The myth emphasizes the suffering resulting from this act. To transcend nature, to be alienated from nature and from another human being, finds man naked, ashamed. He is alone and free, yet powerless and afraid. The newly won freedom appears as a curse; he is free from the sweet bondage of paradise, but he is not free to govern himself, to realize his individuality.[26]

The term "freedom" is employed on seven separate occasions in the text, each instance serving to convey a distinct notion. Fromm's description is meticulously constructed by dialectical logic. A notable element of this analysis is the emphasis on the concept that while an individual is a human being, there is a prohibition against being authentic to oneself. This assertion suggests that, despite being a human being, one is not permitted to be a man. From Fromm's perspective, the individual is a human being, thereby necessitating the cultivation of a human identity. The human being's identity is shaped by the act of sin, which is regarded as the origin of their personal transgressions. It is noteworthy that while the individual has indeed become a human being, he or she has not yet come to recognize his or her "true self." This notion of a "true self" signifies the attainment of self-awareness, which in turn enables the recognition of a positive aspect of one's human nature that has been internalized.

In this foundational context, Fromm expounds on the political implications of freedom. The state of mind in which human beings are unable to accept their own existence has led to constraints imposed by "'secondary bonds' as a substitute for primary bonds which have been lost."[27] This phenomenon, as Fromm articulates, can be conceptualized as a process of "escape from freedom."

> Primary bonds once severed cannot be mended; once paradise is lost, man cannot return to it. There is only one possible, productive solution for the relationship of individualized man with the world: his active solidarity with all men and his spontaneous activity, love and work, which unite him again with the world, not by primary ties but as a free and independent individual. However, if the economic, social and political conditions on which the whole process of human individuation depends, [sic] do not offer a basis for the realization of individuality in the sense just mentioned, while at the same time people have lost those ties which gave them security, *this lag makes freedom an unbearable burden*. It then becomes identical with doubt, with a kind of life which lacks meaning and direction. Powerful tendencies arise to escape from this kind of freedom into submission or some kind of relationship

> to man and the world which promises relief from uncertainty, even if it deprives the individual of his freedom.[28]

From this perspective, societies, to a greater or lesser extent, inherently encompass certain fascist elements. The extent to which a society exhibits fascist tendencies is a critical factor in its classification as fascist or non-fascist.[29] Moreover, an excessive indulgence in narcissistic tendencies has been identified as a pivotal indicator of a society's well-being. According to Fromm's sociopsychological theory, the extent of these characteristics is contingent upon the societal character structure.

Fromm's position is characterized by a persistent assertion that the combination of active love and reason, which he refers to as "productive work," possesses the capacity to liberate individuals from psychological constraints. This liberation, as posited by Fromm, ultimately culminates in the realization of positive freedom and democracy. However, this endeavor appears to be arduous within Fromm's theoretical framework, as he asserts:

> The victory of freedom is possible only if democracy develops into a society in which the individual, his growth and happiness, is the aim and purpose of culture, in which life does not need any justification in success or anything else, and in which the individual is not subordinated to or manipulated by any power outside of himself, be it the State or the economic machine.[30]

## *To Have or To Be?* (1976)

The title of the book *To Have or To Be?* may sound intriguing, but it is precisely about the topic of the book. The term "to have" is defined as the possession of tangible objects, referred to as the "having mode." In contrast, "to be" is interpreted as the appeal to the public, known as the "being mode." The having mode has been identified as a hallmark of "industrial society" and, by extension, the "acquisitive society."[31] The manner in which the being mode functions as "productive activity" is quite distinct from the aforementioned mode of operation:[32] "the mode of existence in which one neither *has* anything nor *craves to have* something, but is joyous, employs one's faculties productively, is *oned* to the world."[33]

The contemporary interpretation of the term "having" is as follows: "to consume is one form of having, and perhaps the most important one for today's affluent industrial societies."[34] Fromm places significant emphasis on the notion that the primary concern in contemporary industrial society is the augmentation of "property," a concept he asserts can be instrumentalized to garner recognition.[35] Fromm posits that, "[t]he nature of the having mode of existence follows from the nature of private property."[36] As previously mentioned, this society subverts the conventional roles of humans and objects, thereby subverting the traditional hierarchical structure. Within this paradigm, the conventional roles of human and object are inverted, resulting in the individual becoming the object and the object becoming the subject. This phenomenon is regarded as a paradox of capitalism, a curious social occurrence that was elucidated by Marx's theory of alienation.

The having mode conceptually encapsulates the prevailing zeitgeist, whereby the preponderance of individuals prioritize the pursuit of consumption over other life priorities. This phenomenon can be characterized as a manifestation of narcissistic tendencies, driven by the desire to indulge in self-centered pleasures. In consideration of these sociocultural factors, contemporary individuals find themselves compelled to prioritize self-promotion and self-consumption in pursuit of objectives that extend beyond mere subsistence. This phenomenon suggests a societal inclination toward a more consumerist lifestyle, where the act of consuming is perceived as a more valuable and meritorious endeavor compared to the pursuit of survival. The pervasive social problem of alienation finds its origins in the capitalist market mechanism, which fosters an environment that prioritizes consumerism. This dynamic perpetuates the ongoing existence of contemporary capitalism.

Furthermore, this underscores the rationale behind Fromm's insistence on the transformation of the having mode into the being mode. In the having mode, characterized by the embodiment of joy, the adept utilization of faculties for productive endeavors, and a profound sense of interconnectedness with the world, individuals find themselves in a state of genuine fulfillment. In light of these elements, contemporary individuals prioritize the realization of their personal needs through the consumption paradigm, while concurrently aligning with societal expectations through a marketing-oriented approach, thereby demonstrating an apt response to the demands of both individual and collective needs. Consequently, the aforementioned elements have a concomitant effect of fortifying the sociostructural framework, thereby engendering a state of disaffection. This, in turn, necessitates an acquiescent stance on the part of the subjects within the prevailing order of market-based capitalism. According to Fromm's theoretical framework, the concept of alienation is posited as a phenomenon that is both reinforced and perpetuated by social structures and the individual, concurrently satisfying their respective needs. This process of internalization entails a systematic adaptation of the individual to the societal environment, thereby engendering a social order irrespective of class distinctions. It is acknowledged that individuals exhibit self-destructive tendencies as a result of their profound passivity in the context of alienation.

### *Human Change*

Fromm's proposal asserts that the achievement of "characterological change" is contingent upon the fulfillment of four criteria by individuals aspiring to this transformation in character structures. These criteria include self-awareness of personal suffering, acknowledgment of the origin of one's "ill-being," recognition of a remedy for one's condition, and understanding of the necessity to modify current living practices in accordance with standards for surmounting adversity.[37] Subsequently, Fromm puts forth the concept of the "new Man," a term denoting an amalgamation of twenty-one qualities concerning the individual's character structures.[38] This concept is posited as a means to establish a "being mode" for the establishment of a new society, one which is founded upon "productive activity." In order to comprehend the significance of understanding Fromm's conceptualization of "human change," it is vital to elucidate the qualities that Fromm asserts are essential for our society. Alongside these societal attributes, the new Man is regarded as a pivotal factor in endowing these qualities, thereby shaping the societal landscape.

Firstly, it is crucial to acknowledge the notion of "willingness" as a fundamental component of the transformation process. The concept of "willingness" is defined as the psychological inclination to transition from the "having mode" to the "being mode." Secondly, the concepts of "security," "sense of identity," and "confidence" are obtained through "relatedness," "interest," "love," and "solidarity" within the being mode. The third principle is the self-acknowledgment of the meaninglessness of one's own life and the self-awareness of "radical independence" and "no-thingness" leading one to "sharing" and "caring." The fourth principle asserts that self-expression is identified as a fundamental aspect of human experience. The fifth principle asserts that satisfaction is derived not from the accumulation and exploitation of material possessions, but from the act of giving and sharing. The sixth principle is defined as the act of "loving" and "respecting" all living creatures. The seventh principle entails the reduction of "greed," "hate," and "illusion." The eighth principle advocates for the avoidance of "worshiping idols" and "illusions." The ninth principle entails the cultivation of the individual's capacity for "love" in conjunction with "critical" thinking. The tenth principle calls for the overcoming of individual "narcissism." The eleventh principle posits the aspiration for the comprehensive evolution of "one's fellow beings." The twelfth principle emphasizes the awareness of the necessity of discipline and respect for reality. The thirteenth principle acknowledges the potential for the flourishing of individuals within the confines of a structured framework, distinguishing between "structure as an attribute of life" and "order as an attribute of no-life, of the dead." The fourteenth principle asserts the necessity of cultivating individual "imagination" to foster expectations for "real possibilities." The fifteenth principle underscores the necessity of abstaining from unethical practices. The sixteenth principle underscores the necessity of self-awareness. The seventeenth principle entails a comprehensive understanding of "nature" and a sense of unity with it. The eighteenth principle asserts that the attainment of personal autonomy is paramount in achieving self-actualization. The nineteenth principle is characterized by a sense of distrust toward "evil" and "destructiveness." The twentieth principle is defined by the absence of "ambition" to fully actualize these two qualities. The twenty-first principle underscores the significance of contentment in oneself, emphasizing the value of ongoing growth and vitality "in the process of ever-growing aliveness."

According to Fromm's theory, the concept of the new Man is inextricably linked to the notion of the new society. A critical aspect of Fromm's theoretical framework is the prioritization of the formation of a new Man over the establishment of a new society. This suggests that the transformation of individual characters precedes the structural transformation of society. In addressing potential solutions to social challenges, Fromm proposes specific modifications to contemporary society.

Firstly, it is imperative to reconstruct the "industrial mode of production without total centralization." Secondly, the decentralization of planning and the abolition of the "free-market economy" are essential components of this approach. Thirdly, the objective of this approach is not the pursuit of unlimited growth, but rather the cultivation of selective growth. Fourthly, the establishment of working conditions conducive to spiritual motivation is also paramount. Fifthly, the development of science must be undertaken in a manner that does not pose a threat to the well-being of humanity. Sixthly, the establishment of social conditions conducive to well-being is necessary. Seventhly, ensuring the fundamental security of individuals and their autonomy is of paramount importance. Finally, the realization of "individual initiative in living" is imperative.

In consideration of the aforementioned criteria, it is reasonable to conclude that the probability of establishing a new Man or a new society is minimal. Fromm advances a viewpoint on this matter, and while I do not contest his perspective, further examination is necessary to fully understand its implications. While the realization of these criteria would undoubtedly be arduous, even seemingly futile, it is by no means unfeasible. Fromm is keenly cognizant of the limitations of his perspective (2011 [1976]: 159). He acknowledges the challenges involved, yet he remains steadfast in his commitment to these efforts, channeling all his energy into the task, despite the daunting odds of success. From a psychoanalytic perspective, Fromm's adoption of a more challenging approach to societal transformation, as evidenced by his conceptualization of a new society, can be understood as a pragmatic conclusion that contemporary society, as he perceived it, necessitated a more efficacious intervention. This remedy, he posits, must enable society to confront its own unconscious through therapeutic praxis, thereby curing its narcissistic ailment.

## Notes

1 Funk, *Das Leben selbst ist eine Kunst*, 72.
2 Erich Fromm, *Das jüdische Gesetz: Zur Soziologie des Diaspora-Judentums. Schriften aus dem Nachlaß, Band 2*, Rainer Funk (Ed.) (Weinheim und Basel: Beltz Verlag, 1989 [1922]).

3 Chad Kautzer, "Marx's Influence on the Early Frankfurt School," in Michael J. Thompson (Ed.), *The Palgrave Handbook of Critical Theory* (New York: Palgrave Macmillan, 2017), 43–66.
4 Erich Fromm, *Escape from Freedom* (New York: Rinehart and Company, 1941), 270.
5 Fromm, *Escape from Freedom*, 270.
6 Only *Beyond the Chains of Illusion* (1962) and *Social Character in a Mexican Village* (1970), two of the more than 20 books published since *Escape from Freedom*, have seriously addressed and examined this concept. The latter, however, is rather different in that it is an empirical study to test the validity of the concept of "social character."
7 However, the outcomes of Adorno's empirical social psychological research in the mid-1960s, in which he inherited Fromm's concept of the "authoritarian personality," can be substantiated through historical evidence in the domain of social and political psychology. Consequently, Fromm's contributions to the field of social psychology are indisputable.
8 See, e.g., Grey, "Society as Destiny"; Takamichi Sakurai, *Political Theories of Narcissism: Towards Self-Reflection on Knowledge and Politics from the Psychoanalytic Perspectives of Erich Fromm and Fujita Shōzō* (Zürich: LIT Verlag, 2018), 217.
9 Salvador Millán, "The Social Dimensions of Transference," Paper for the Erich Fromm International Symposium, Washington, DC, 8 May 1994. Retrieved from: http://opus4.kobv.de/opus4-Fromm/files/16525/Millan_S_1992.pdf, 1–7, at 5.
10 Fromm, *Escape from Freedom*, 141.
11 Fromm, *Escape from Freedom*, 36.
12 Fromm, *Escape from Freedom*, 36–37.
13 Erich Fromm, *The Anatomy of Human Destructiveness*, 1st ed. (New York: Henry Holt & Company. 1992 [1973]), 325.
14 Fromm, *The Anatomy of Human Destructiveness*, 325.
15 Fromm, *The Anatomy of Human Destructiveness*, 330–32.
16 Fromm, *The Anatomy of Human Destructiveness*, 338.
17 Fromm, *The Anatomy of Human Destructiveness*, 339.
18 Fromm, *The Anatomy of Human Destructiveness*, 339.
19 Fromm, *The Anatomy of Human Destructiveness*, 280–324.
20 Fromm, *Escape from Freedom*, 22–23; Fromm, *Man for Himself*, 45.
21 Fromm *Escape from Freedom*, 22–23.
22 Indeed, the term "dialectic" has been referenced in the context of Fromm's political perspective. This is particularly evident in the notion that freedom undergoes a dialectical process (e.g., Stephen E. Bronner, "Fromm in America," in Michael Kessler and Rainer Funk (Eds), *Erich Fromm und die Frankfurter Schule* (Tübingen: Francke Verlag, 1992), 41–59; Ramon Xirau, "Erich Fromm: What Is Man's Struggle?," in Bernard Landis and Edward S. Tauber (Eds), *In the Name of Life: Essays in Honor of Erich Fromm* (New York: Holt, Rinehart & Winston, 1971), 150–60; cf. Fromm, *Escape from Freedom*, 35, 104). Moreover, the term is salient in relation to Fromm's perspective on human nature, particularly concerning his conception of "dichotomies" (e.g., Joan Braune, "Erich Fromm and Thomas Merton: Biophilia, Necrophilia, and Messianism," *Fromm Forum* (English version), 15 (2011): 43–48; Marianne Horney Eckardt, "Fromm's Humanistic Ethics and the Role of the Prophet," in Mauricio Cortina and Michael Maccoby (Eds), *A Prophetic Analyst: Erich Fromm's Contribution to Psychoanalysis* (Northvale and London: Jason Aronson, 1996), 151–66; Millán, "The Social Dimensions of Transference").

23 See, e.g., Neil McLaughlin, "Nazism, Nationalism, and the Sociology of Emotions: *Escape from Freedom* Revisited," *Sociological Theory*, 14, no. 3 (1996): 241–61.
24 This scholarly connection has been extensively explored in various academic works, including those by Kessler and Funk, *Erich Fromm und die Frankfurter Schule* and Joel Whitebook, "Fantasy and Critique: Some Thoughts on Freud and the Frankfurt School," in David M. Rasmusssen (Ed.), *The Handbook of Critical Theory* (Oxford: Blackwell, 1996), 287–304, at 288.
25 Fromm, *Escape from Freedom*, 32.
26 Fromm, *Escape from Freedom*, 33–35; emphases added.
27 Fromm, *Escape from Freedom*, 141.
28 Fromm, *Escape from Freedom*, 36–37; emphases added.
29 This issue pertains to the sociological and sociopsychological discourses surrounding the concept of fascism. In the context of Fromm's theoretical framework, the concept of fascism is directed not only toward describing so-called Fascism, depicted in certain periods of time in history. Instead, the crux of his social theory lies in its conceptualization of fascism as a pathological phenomenon of alienation. This theoretical framework posits that human beings become commodities subject to capital, thereby losing their inherent autonomy and suppressing their intrinsic, positive human nature. This theoretical perspective is characterized by its emphasis on the complete absorption of individuals into the system of administration. From Fromm's perspective, the hallmark of fascism lies in the extent to which individuals adopt a bureaucratic approach to their own social conduct. This viewpoint is further elaborated upon in his assertion that bureaucrats who adopt a rigid, systematic approach are more perilous than those who adhere to a fanatical fascist ideology (Fromm, *To Have or To Be?*, 151–52).
30 Fromm, *Escape from Freedom*, 270–71.
31 Fromm, *To Have or To Be?* 57.
32 Fromm, *To Have or To Be?* e.g., 74.
33 Fromm, *To Have or To Be?* 16.
34 Fromm, *To Have or To Be?* 23.
35 Fromm, *To Have or To Be?* 58.
36 Fromm, *To Have or To Be?* 63.
37 Fromm, *To Have or To Be?* 137.
38 Fromm, *To Have or To Be?* 139–40.

# 2 Fromm's Main Theoretical Contribution

## Fromm's Psychoanalytic Theory

Fromm's initial encounter with psychoanalysis occurred during his Heidelberg years in the 1920s. It is widely accepted that his psychoanalysis was initiated by his encounter with Frieda Fromm-Reichmann, a psychiatrist who would subsequently become his spouse.[1] Fromm's 1926 marriage to Reichmann symbolized this event. The couple's joint establishment of the Institute for Psychoanalysis at the University of Berlin in 1929 further solidified their position as prominent figures in the field.

While Fromm's social and critical theorizing in the 1920s remains challenging to fully apprehend, it is in this period that we may commence to discern the spiritual underpinnings of his oeuvre. A seminal example of the integration of psychoanalysis and sociology can be found in his 1929 work, "Psychoanalysis and Sociology." Concurrently, the evidence suggests that he was engaged in psychoanalysis. These facts are crucial to understanding Fromm because psychoanalysis undoubtedly plays a central role in his theoretical framework. In particular, Fromm's psychoanalytic theory, which emphasizes the detrimental effects of the "market mentality," unveils unsettling realities about contemporary market society, as noted by the psychoanalyst Ruth Lesser.[2] In essence, Fromm's perspective posits that psychoanalysis functions as the foundational basis for the "immanent critique," which he deems to be the most substantial element of critical theory.[3]

However, as previously mentioned in the Introduction, Fromm's psychoanalysis has historically encountered a lack of serious consideration within the mainstream psychoanalytic discourse. This assertion is particularly salient in the context of his theory of narcissism. For instance, Fromm is mentioned only once in *The Handbook of Narcissism and Narcissistic Personality Disorder* (2011).[4] The eminent theorist of narcissism, Elsa Ronningstam, does not even mention Fromm's contribution in her seminal work, *Identifying and Understanding Narcissistic Personality* (2005).[5] As demonstrated by the aforementioned facts, it can be posited that Fromm's theory of narcissism has remained outside the ambit of psychoanalysis.

In contrast, it is evident that Fromm's psychoanalysis has garnered a measure of acknowledgment. The following four perspectives can be used to

DOI: 10.4324/9781003600398-3

summarize the evaluation of his psychoanalysis:[6] first, a direct contribution to psychoanalysis (in Fromm's "analytic social psychology" method and in the concepts of "social transference" and "mental health"); second, a contribution to the theoretical foundations of the social sciences within his theory of "social character"; third, an evaluation of the ethical implications of his humanistic theory of ethics for clinical practice; and fourth, the theoretical and therapeutic implications of Fromm's theory of narcissism for psychoanalysis. This distinguishing characteristic of this perspective is its utilization of a "social" framework to mediate these assessments. In summary, Fromm's psychoanalysis is predicated on the integration of psychoanalysis with the social sciences. However, as has been previously noted, his interdisciplinary endeavors have historically been overlooked.

Fromm scholars who favor Fromm's psychoanalysis have noted that it is critical of traditional psychoanalytic approaches and offers a way out by attributing "social determinants" to psychoanalysis.[7] However, the evaluation of Fromm's psychoanalysis is predominantly influenced by one's methodological approach, that is to say, the academic discipline and school of thought from which one interprets his psychoanalytical concepts. For instance, while Fromm's psychoanalysis undoubtedly possesses the aforementioned advantages, it can be perceived negatively by psychoanalysts and clinical psychologists, whose position is that the most crucial aspect is the commitment to the treatment of the individual. In this regard, it is essential to acknowledge that Fromm's perspective is not unassailable. While the role of "social determinants" in influencing human mental activity is indeed significant, this does not imply an absolute nature of this influence. Despite the underappreciated status of Fromm's psychoanalysis within the psychoanalytic community, it is crucial to underscore that any deliberate or inadvertent absolutization or deification of his position would, paradoxically, serve to subvert his endeavors.

As previously stated, the true appeal of Fromm's psychoanalysis resides in its interconnection with social issues. For this reason, his psychoanalysis is designated as "sociological psychoanalysis."[8] This manifests at the social level, as evidenced by the attribution of a sociological function to psychoanalysis, a topic that will be explored below.[9] First and foremost, this facilitates the identification of *social* pathologies.

The central question guiding this inquiry is to ascertain the most significant aspects of Fromm's psychoanalysis. This phenomenon can be interpreted as a search for spiritual sustenance within the context of societal engagement. This approach has the potential to enhance both the societal fabric and the social life of individuals. Fromm's psychoanalysis, however, is primarily prescriptive from a self-reflective perspective, pointing to the locus of society's spiritual problems. This is due to the fact that, as will be discussed subsequently, its ultimate objective is the *healing of society*. This underscores the necessity of adopting a critical theory perspective and further emphasizes the importance of psychoanalysis in comprehending the intricacies of human behavior.

In light of the aforementioned examination, the following three main features of Fromm's psychoanalysis are evident.

Firstly, it underscores the significance of "social determinants" in the context of human spiritual life. As previously mentioned, this may be perceived as an indication of Fromm's academic bias, given that it is a definitive articulation of the fact that his psychoanalysis is specifically directed toward the analysis of society. While this assertion is undoubtedly valid to a certain extent, it is imperative to acknowledge that this perspective overlooks a crucial element. This standpoint is consistent with the predominant tenets of Fromm and Freudian psychoanalysis, which postulate that the individual is inherently intertwined with their environment. In particular, Fromm's "social need" is a concept that provides a coherent explanation for this phenomenon.

Secondly, Fromm employs a transdisciplinary approach by integrating psychoanalysis with the social sciences, thereby extending the conceptual framework of the former to the latter. This approach enables the utilization of psychiatric and psychoanalytic epistemology and methodology in the *examination*, *diagnosis*, and *treatment* of society within the domain of the social sciences. This self-reflective perspective is characterized by introspection and is cultivated through a reciprocal human interaction between the therapist (analyst) and the treated (patient). This approach has the potential to address the limitations of traditional social sciences, which often exhibit one-sidedness in their methodologies.

Thirdly, Fromm's psychoanalysis elucidates the ideology of market capitalism by underscoring the deleterious effects of the "marketplace mentality" on the human psyche. The cornerstone of our societal structure is predicated on the exchange of goods within the marketplace, wherein individuals assume the role of consumers in relation to the items they procure. Fromm's argument is that the market economy is inherently detrimental to society and must be abandoned. Fromm's psychoanalysis renders his position sui generis.

As previously mentioned, Fromm's psychoanalytic approach encompasses a comprehensive examination of "society" in its myriad facets, with the entity of "society" itself serving as the focal point of analysis. For this reason, Fromm's psychoanalysis has the potential to not only enhance the field of social sciences through its epistemological and methodological contributions, but also to benefit society in a pragmatic manner. However, it is crucial to refrain from an uncritical acceptance of Fromm's perspective. Instead, there is a necessity to maintain a degree of flexibility and adaptability, making adjustments as circumstances demand—this approach is not confined solely to the realm of psychoanalysis but extends to various fields of study and practice.

### Authoritarianism

Fromm first formulated his theory of authoritarianism in the early Frankfurt School treatise, *Studien über Autorität und Familie* (Studies on Authority and Family) (1936).[10] However, the scope of his responsibilities in this particular work is rather constrained. Fromm's analysis of the role of the father, as it pertains to German bourgeois and middle-class families, is centered on the emergence of authoritarianism at the social level. Fromm proffers two perspectives on authoritarianism. First, he contends that the Western patriarchal family system has played a role in fostering an authoritarian dynamic among fathers within two different dimensions: the home and the nation. Consequently, this dynamic led to the conferral of patriarchal authority within the latter dimension. Second, Fromm proposes that authoritarianism is initially manifested within the family sphere, acting as a mediator between society and the individual. Fromm's foundational contributions to the field are marked by his seminal research, particularly his identification of the sociopsychological underpinnings and origins of authoritarianism within the context of family. This theoretical framework notably intertwines the examination of authoritarianism within the family unit with its manifestation at the social level, offering a nuanced and integrated understanding of the phenomenon. According to the findings of the aforementioned sociopsychological work, Fromm proceeded to further develop his theory of authoritarianism in *Escape from Freedom* (1941) by examining the sociopsychological underpinnings of Nazism from a psychoanalytic perspective, with a particular focus on the relationship between "sadomasochism" and the political ideology.[11]

Fromm's argument posits that the pathological phenomenon of sadomasochistic symbiosis is a hallmark of the authoritarian personality structure that underlies fascist politics. According to Fromm, within the context of this symbiotic human relationship, individuals develop sadomasochistic desires due to a pathological interdependence, which arises from the unbearable pain experienced in the context of loneliness. This social condition is attributed to the atomization of the individual and the emergence of mass society. Sadomasochism, says Fromm, constitutes the primary factor in a sociopathological dynamic, wherein individuals are compelled to form attachments to a "secondary bond."[12] He argues that an alternative to the "primary bonds" from which people are independent functions as a means of escaping the psychological state of loneliness, regardless of the loss of freedom. This, in turn, serves to bind individuals together under the umbrella of mass social conditions.[13] The following assertions have been made by Fromm:

> Primary bonds once severed cannot be mended; once paradise is lost, man cannot return to it. There is only one possible, productive solution for the relationship of individualized man with the world: his active solidarity with all men and his spontaneous activity, love and work, which unite him again with the world, not by primary ties but as a

> free and independent individual. However, if the economic, social and political conditions on which the whole process of human individuation depends, [sic] do not offer a basis for the realization of individuality in the sense just mentioned, while at the same time people have lost those ties which gave them security, this lag makes freedom an unbearable burden. It then becomes identical with doubt, with a kind of life which lacks meaning and direction. Powerful tendencies arise to escape from this kind of freedom into submission or some kind of relationship to man and the world which promises relief from uncertainty, even if it deprives the individual of his freedom.[14]

As Fromm articulates, "his active solidarity with all men and his spontaneous activity, love and work...unite him again with the world, not by primary ties but as a free and independent individual." In Fromm's social theory, the concept of an incestuous bond that serves to bind people together functions pathologically in an authoritarian way that simultaneously indulges both the sadistic desire to gain control over people as subordinates and the masochistic desire to become powerful by transferring one's weak psychology to authority as superior to the seizure of power itself—Fromm's theory posits that these elements and their very raison d'être are essentially interdependent. Specifically, individuals characterized by sadism and masochism exhibit a tendency toward authoritarianism, as defined by Fromm's theoretical framework. As Fromm argues, fascist politics predicated on sadomasochistic authoritarianism emanate from "[p]owerful tendencies ...to escape from... freedom into submission or some kind of relationship to man and the world which promises relief from uncertainty."

In his subsequent work, *The Anatomy of Human Destructiveness* (1973), Fromm advanced his theory of authoritarianism in clinical, pathological terms.[15] A notable aspect of this work is the application of the concept of necrophilia to the discourse on fascism. According to Fromm, necrophilia is defined as the "love of the dead," which is theoretically classified into two distinct categories: the term "sexual necrophilia" refers to a "man's desire to have sexual intercourse or any other kind of sexual contact with a female corpse," while "nonsexual necrophilia" denotes the "desire to handle, to be near to, and to gaze at corpses, and particularly the desire to disremember them."[16] In this book, I explore how Fromm employs the concept of necrophilia to establish a link between his pathological and characterological theories. He delineates the "necrophilous character" as a "passionate attraction to all that is dead, decayed, putrid, sickly," citing the German criminal psychologist Hans von Hentig.[17] Fromm states as follows:

> it is the passion to transform that which is alive into something unalive; to destroy for the sake of destruction; the exclusive interest in all that is purely mechanical. It is the passion "to tear apart living structures."[18]

In particular, Fromm's analysis of Hitler's necrophilous tendencies is particularly noteworthy. A prime example of this tendency is Adolf Hitler, who, according to the extant literature, was driven by a penchant for necrophilia, as evidenced by his desire to "transform a man into a corpse."[19] According to Fromm, individuals with a necrophilous orientation, such as Hitler, demonstrate a proclivity for the extermination of all things by force. As Fromm articulates, "[w]hat has been, i.e. what is dead, rules his life: institutions, laws, property, traditions, and possessions." Consequently, "things rule man; having rules being; the dead rule the living."[20] In this context, there is an absence of tangible entities, both human and non-human. Instead, abstract entities exist as a means of force. From this perspective, necrophilia is characterized by destruction. A destructive aspect of the character is associated with "sadism," i.e., authoritarianism.[21] Notably, Fromm has provided a pathological, clinical concept for a political analysis of fascism. In essence, Fromm's work aims to illuminate the essence of authoritarianism by exploring its sociopathological underpinnings, a concept he has developed through the lens of psychoanalysis. In doing so, he seeks to elucidate the sociopsychological basis of Nazism.

## Alienation

Fromm's theoretical framework is predominantly influenced by Marx's philosophical contributions, particularly his conception of alienation and its theoretical implications.[22] According to Marx, alienation constitutes a sociopathological phenomenon wherein individuals are regarded as objects of capital within the capitalist system. In this social state, individuals experience profound psychological distress due to their compulsion to adopt a predominantly passive lifestyle. In other words, they become "labor power" that merely generates "surplus value."[23] As Marx asserts:

> alienated labor turns the species-life of man, and also nature as his mental species-property, into an alien being and into a means for his individual existence. It alienates from man his own body, external nature, his mental life and his human life … A direct consequence of the alienation of man from the product of his labor, from his life activity and from his species life is that man is alienated from other men. When man confronts himself he also confronts other men. What is true of man's relationship to his work, to the product of his work and to himself, is also true of his relationship to other men, to their labor and to the objects of their labor. In general, the statement that man is alienated from his species life means that each man is alienated from others, and that each of the others is likewise alienated from human life.[24]

Utilizing his own conception of "marketing orientation," Fromm fleshes out Marx's theory of alienation.[25] In Fromm's theoretical scheme, the marketing orientation is conceptualized as a character structure that has emerged in the modern age as a "modern product" that fulfills the "economic function of the market."[26] This phenomenon indicates a discernible shift in the prevailing character structure, a consequence of the dynamic adaptation of individuals to the prevailing market mechanisms inherent in a capitalist system. The central theoretical implication of the marketing orientation can be expressed as follows: "I am as you desire me."[27] As Fromm puts it, "what matters is ... his [a marketing-oriented person's] success in the process of selling them [commodities]" and "the experience of oneself as a commodity and of one's value as exchange value."[28] The fundamental principle underlying this concept is the act of selling oneself as labor power, that is, as wage labor. In essence, the human being has been reduced to a socioeconomic function of capital, which affects the entire scope of human life. As such, the marketing orientation has evolved into a pivotal component of contemporary identity.

Moreover, the marketing orientation is found to be significantly influenced by Fromm's distinctive concept of "having mode."[29] It is believed that these concepts are inspired by the philosophical contributions of Marx and Meister Eckhart. In this perspective, the "having mode" serves as a counter-concept to the "being mode."[30] According to Fromm, the having mode is a hallmark feature of industrial society, which he refers to as the "acquisitive society."[31] As Fromm phrases it, "[t]he nature of the having mode of existence follows from the nature of private property,"[32] and concomitantly, "to consume is one form of having, and perhaps the most important one for today's affluent industrial societies."[33] The having mode, in essence, encapsulates the prevailing zeitgeist, wherein the preponderance of individuals prioritize the gratification of their own egotistical inclinations through the pursuit of material acquisitions. From this perspective, within the context of contemporary social conditions, individuals appear to prioritize the pursuit of self-sale not solely for the purpose of survival, but also as a means of attaining consumer goods—this inclination suggests that the latter aspect is increasingly deemed a more significant aspect of life in contemporary society. As a result, the problematic social condition of alienation remains constant. The foundation of contemporary capitalism is the capitalist market mechanism, which fosters an environment conducive to consumption. Fromm's argument is compelling. He asserts that this paradigm shift from the "having mode" to the "being mode" is imperative, characterizing the latter as a state of being characterized as "one is joyous, employs one's faculties productively, [and] is oned to the world."[34]

In contemporary society, individuals prioritize the satisfaction of their personal needs through the pursuit of material possessions, while simultaneously aligning with societal expectations through a marketing-oriented approach, thereby catering to both individual and collective desires. As a result, they contribute to the reinforcement of a sociocharacter structure that induces alienation and requires them to assume a passive role in the system of market capitalism. In Fromm's view, alienation is perpetuated and its social condition is regenerated by both society and the individual. Both fulfill their respective desires, with the latter adapting to the former and internalizing its needs, regardless of social class. According to Fromm's theoretical framework, individuals manifest self-destructive tendencies due to their passive position in the face of alienation. Updating Marx's conception of alienation, Fromm sought to demonstrate that "the clerk, the salesman, the executive, are even more alienated today than the skilled manual worker," and that "as far as consumption is concerned, there is no difference between manual workers and the members of the bureaucracy."[35]

## Narcissism

The issues inherent in Fromm's theory of narcissism remain unaddressed, even within the confines of Fromm research. Moreover, as previously mentioned, mainstream psychoanalysis has predominantly disregarded this facet. The predominant rationale for this oversight can be attributed to the "cross-disciplinary, multi-layered structure of the theory." This interdisciplinary framework encompasses psychoanalytic and sociotheoretical concepts, a complexity that often perplexes contemporary scholars confined to a single-disciplinary domain.[36] Apart from this, the disregard is, at least in part, attributable to the robust emphasis placed on the "negative impact of the marketplace mentality" on human psychology in Fromm's psychoanalytic theory.[37]

Despite this unfavorable reputation, Fromm scholars, including psychoanalysts, acknowledge the merit of his conception of narcissism.[38] Marco Bacciagaluppi (1993) underscores its pertinence across three domains: theoretical, sociopathological, and clinical. In Fromm's social theory, narcissism is conceptualized as a "character structure" within the sociopathological realm.[39] In this context, Fromm draws parallels between narcissism and market society, juxtaposing the two according to their respective social functions. This linkage, however, is the source of the perplexities of his theory of narcissism and his psychoanalytic theory. As previously mentioned, these perplexities have been the object of scorn by contemporary researchers in various disciplinary fields, as well as by psychoanalysts in general. In other words, the theoretical underpinnings of his psychoanalytic theory have been deemed to exceed the scope of conventional academic disciplines, a consequence of its comprehensive interdisciplinary conflation.

### *Narcissism as Selfishness: A Psychoanalytic Concept*

Freud is the source of Fromm's conception of narcissism. Freud's following definition is arguably most pertinent to Fromm: "[n]arcissism . . . would not be a perversion, but the libidinal complement to the egoism of the instinct of self-preservation, a measure of which may justifiably be attributed to every living creature."[40] This shift in perspective potentially had a substantial impact on Fromm's theoretical scheme, prompting him to conceptualize narcissism in terms of egoism, particularly "selfishness."[41] As will be demonstrated in the following section, however, Fromm advanced a perspective that stands in stark contrast to Freud's. Fromm asserted that self-love constitutes an integral component of the concept of love, whereas narcissism is counterproductive to this self-love.[42]

Fromm conceptualizes narcissism as a form of "selfishness," characterized by the withdrawal of love from others and its reorientation toward the self.[43] In his perspective, the capacity to love others and oneself is impeded by one's inclination toward self-centeredness, which is distinct from the concept of "self-love."[44] This is often characterized in the following manner, as articulated by Fromm: "While on the surface it seems that [narcissistic] persons are very much in love with themselves, they actually are not fond of themselves, and their narcissism—like selfishness—is an overcompensation for the basic lack of self-love."[45] Fromm expounds on the underlying cause of this fundamental deficit as follows.

> Narcissism can then be described as a state of experience in which only the person himself, his body, his needs, his feelings, his thoughts, his property, everything and everybody pertaining to him are experienced as fully real, while everybody and everything that does not form part of the person or is not an object of his needs is not interesting, is not fully real, is perceived only by intellectual recognition, while affectively without weight and color.[46]

From this perspective, Fromm concludes: "[s]*elfishness and self-love, far from being identical, are actually opposites*."[47] As a result of this reflection, his perspective on narcissism is predominantly critical from a humanist perspective.

### *Benign and Malignant Narcissism: A Pathological Concept*

Fromm's dialectical perspective extends beyond psychoanalysis, observing narcissism as pathological in both benign and malignant forms.[48] The most compelling illustration of this dialectical mechanism is the phenomenon that an illness, whether physical or mental, often exhibits periods of fluctuation between positive and negative phases. In pathological terms, Fromm goes on to define the benign form as "self-checking" and the malignant form as "not self-limiting."[49] As he articulates it, "[i]n the benign form the object of narcissism is the result of a person's effort," while "[i]n the case of malignant narcissism, [it] is not anything the person does or produces, but something he *has* …" It "is not self-limiting, and in consequence … crudely solipsistic as well as xenophobic."[50] The most malignant type is predicted to engender far-right politics characterized by ethnonationalism and xenophobia.

### *Social Narcissism: A Sociological Concept*

Moreover, Fromm divides narcissism into two kinds according to what he calls "biological and sociological functions": individual narcissism and social narcissism—he often substitutes "group narcissism" for the latter.[51] Fromm's theoretical framework enables the quantitative analysis of this discrepancy, thereby demonstrating the former manifestation of narcissism as being *analogous* to the latter.[52] In summary, the two phenomena under discussion are distinct in terms of their respective quantitative characteristics, as evidenced by the divergent findings in the domains of individual and social psychology.[53] This is a crucial feature of Fromm's psychoanalytic theory. The quantitative difference inherent in both psychology and social psychology allows Fromm to identify both individual and social illnesses. This observation lends support to the notion that Fromm's emphasis on the narcissistic orientation, particularly in the context of social narcissism, is a deliberate and well-considered approach. Indeed, he is regarded not only as a psychoanalyst but also as a "sociological psychoanalyst."[54] Fromm himself demonstrated this in a provocative sociological integration of Freud's psychoanalysis with Marx's historical materialism in his pioneering 1932 essay "The Method and Function of an Analytic Social Psychology."[55]

### *Group Narcissism: The Pathological Development of Politics*

The concept of "group narcissism" is a product of Fromm's sociopsychological method, which has its roots in psychoanalysis.[56] The assumption is that it is to some extent related to aggression and therefore has a pathological dimension. Fromm asserts that this phenomenon constitutes "one of the most important sources of human aggression, and yet this, like all other forms of defensive aggression, is a reaction to an attack on vital interests."[57] In fact, Fromm contends that malignant or extreme narcissism fosters wanton destruction, citing Adolf Hitler and Heinrich Himmler as exemplars.[58]

Group narcissism manifests in three distinct ways: firstly, in the "narcissistic cathexis"; secondly, in the dialectical, developmental process of benign and malignant narcissism; and thirdly, in the realm of malignant group gratification.[59] The preliminary notion concerns the process by which constituents impart to a collective with energies that can be categorized as either benign or malignant narcissism. This phenomenon enables the group to function effectively in response to anger. Fromm's account offers a compelling exposition of the phenomenon of group narcissism. He posits that it becomes "compatible with social co-operation" when its needs are benignly directed toward productive activity. Conversely, he asserts that "narcissistic passion" emerges when these needs are absorbed in a malignant manner within the "splendor" of a group, "its past achievements," and the "physique of its members."[60] The third approach elucidates the underlying rationales for the pervasive support of extreme forms of narcissism, such as political fanaticism, chauvinism, and ethnonationalism, which are invariably heavily supported by the pursuit of malignant narcissistic gratification. This phenomenon can be attributed to the fact that it represents the sole source of contentment for the group members.

The mechanisms of group narcissism are reinforced by those of individual narcissism. The phenomenon of individual narcissism operates through the provision of individual narcissistic energy to a group. However, within Fromm's theoretical framework, narcissism frequently evolves into a form of social malady. Thus, the pathological functions of narcissism should be the primary focus when addressing group narcissism issues—this underscores the relevance of the second and third pathways that are highly relevant to group narcissism from a sociopathological perspective. Specifically, Fromm emphasizes the four characteristics of pathological group narcissism: a "lack of objectivity and rational judgement," the necessity of "narcissistic satisfaction," a "reaction of rage," and narcissistic "symbiosis and identification."[61] Narcissism has been demonstrated to be *pathologically* associated with politics, as will be further elaborated upon in the following discussion. This phenomenon, as articulated by Fromm, is primarily attributable to the fact that "[in]asmuch as the group as a whole requires group narcissism for its survival, it will further narcissistic attitudes and confer upon them the qualification of being particularly virtuous."[62] Put simply, a group type of narcissism is compelled to adopt an increasingly narcissistic disposition, as it requires the cathexis of individual narcissism to maintain its vitality. In accordance with Fromm's theoretical framework, the mechanisms of group narcissism function predominantly through the medium of malignant group satisfaction. This can be attributed to the dialectic relationship between benign and malignant narcissism, which is often influenced by pathological political movements such as ethnonationalism and chauvinism. These movements frequently gain traction within the social context of market capitalism, where individuals experience an overwhelming need for narcissistic gratification. In the prevailing interpretation of Fromm's theoretical scheme, it is arguable that the emergence of such movements within the context of an authoritarian sociocharacter structure may result in the adoption of fascist political ideologies. Irrespective of this, the capitalist market society hinges upon the mechanisms of narcissism and the character structure of its society. This underscores the notion that the fundamental purpose of these individuals is predicated solely on their own narcissistic proclivities, thereby propelling the market economy to operate in its current state.

As previously mentioned, it is possible to observe the development of fascist politics within the theoretical scheme of Fromm's theory of narcissism. According to Fromm's political formulation of narcissism, "[g]roup narcissism is a phenomenon of the greatest political significance." He further asserts that "if he [a narcissist] can identify with his nation, or can transfer his personal narcissism to the nation, then he is everything" and thus becomes omnipotent by finding himself a "member of the most wonderful group on earth"—these views are integral to Fromm's political theory of narcissism.[63] According to Fromm, a malignant type of group narcissism essentially threatens to provoke political behavior associated with "fanaticism" and "destructiveness" because it is characterized by a lack of self-control, including that of objectivity and rational judgment, and by a sense of total power that makes a person feel like he or she is all things to all people—in fact, Fromm sees an uncontrolled state of mind and sadistic omnipotence as major factors in these two pathologies.[64] This dynamic suggests a transfer of the malignant narcissistic need to "nation," "race," "religion," and other constructs, thereby giving rise to political fanaticism.[65] Fromm argues:

> If … [a] narcissistically inflated group does not have available a minority which is sufficiently helpless to lend itself as an object for narcissistic satisfaction, the group's narcissism will easily lead to the wish for military conquests; this was the path of pan-Germanism and pan-Slav ism before 1914. In both cases the respective nations were endowed with the role of being the "chosen nation," superior to all others, and hence justified in attacking those who did not accept their superiority… their fanaticism was certainly one factor which contributed to the outbreak of the war. Beyond this, however, one must not forget that once a war has started, the various governments try to arouse national narcissism as a necessary psychological condition for the successful waging of the war.[66]

Although Fromm refrains from using the term "fascism" in this context, a combination of narcissistic, necrophilous, and sadomasochistic character structures emerges clearly in Fromm's theoretical framework as the socio-psychological basis of fascism: the "syndrome of decay."[67] In other words, Fromm proposes that narcissism is a contributing factor in the rise of fascist politics, though he does not inherently define fascism within the framework of his characterological theory. Indeed, it is argued that, in his subsequent years, he arrived at the conclusion that the provenance of fascist political orientations is not, in fact, rooted in authoritarianism predicated on sadomasochism.[68] Additionally, a specific facet of fascist ideologies can be illuminated through the prism of Western Marxism, particularly the concept of the "dialectic of enlightenment."[69] This concept posits that fascist ideologies represent a contradiction within economic rationality. Moreover, it is noteworthy that even in the postwar period, there have been sufficient sociopathological milieux in which people have nurtured the desire to depend exclusively on authoritative affiliations such as nation, race, and religion in the context of mass society. It is evident that these conditions are accompanied by narcissism. These issues are of particular importance in the sense that contemporary market-oriented society is structured by a narcissistic orientation, as in Fromm's social theory.[70] Narcissism exerts a pervasive influence on human life, particularly in contexts characterized by the values of "separateness and antagonism of individuals toward each other" and the "worship of industrial production." It can be argued that these elements serve as fundamental conditions that facilitate the proliferation of narcissism.[71] Group narcissism has been observed to flourish in the context of contemporary mass society, as

> [a] highly narcissistic group is eager to have a leader with whom it can identify itself. The leader is then admired by the group which projects its narcissism onto him. In the very act of submission to the powerful leader, which is in depth an act of symbiosis and identification, the narcissism of the individual is transferred onto the leader. The greater the leader, the greater the follower. Personalities who as individuals are particularly narcissistic are the most qualified to fulfil this function. The narcissism of the leader who is convinced of his greatness, and who has no doubts, is precisely what attracts the narcissism of those who submit to him. The half-insane leader is often the most successful one until his lack of objective judgement, his rage reactions in consequence of any set-back, his need to keep up the image of omnipotence may provoke him to make mistakes which lead to his destruction. But there are always gifted half-psychotics at hand to satisfy the demands of a narcissistic mass.[72]

A similar phenomenon occurs in the context of contemporary mass society, where narcissism is employed to formulate a pathological politics characterized by alienation and isolation. The emergence of fascist politics is a plausible outcome of these conditions.[73] This phenomenon, as elucidated by Fromm, underscores the notion that fascism can thrive even in the absence of an authoritarian character structure.

### Fascism

The term "fascism" is derived from the Italian word "fascio," which means a "bundle of rods," and is a sign of strong group solidarity.[74] This observation indicates that fascism initially flourished within the Italian political landscape.[75] In the sense of its emergence in 1919, it is distinct from long-standing political phenomena such as traditional autocracy, despotism, dictatorship, and tyranny, whose conceptual implications overlap with those of fascism. Conceptually, the term "fascism" is used to denote a "generalized historical type of authoritarian political regime."[76] According to Roger Griffin, a preeminent theorist of fascism, the term can be defined as a "revolutionary form of ultranationalism that attempts to realize the myth of the regenerated nation."[77] From this fundamental definition, he proceeds to explore the nature of fascism:

> It is a myth which applied in practice creates a totalitarian movement or regime engaged in combating cultural, ethnic and even biological ("dysgenic") decadence and engineering a new sort of "man" in an alternative socio-political and cultural modernity to liberal capitalism.[78]

According to Griffin, fascism is an alternative to "liberal capitalism" and is based on a nationalist ideology that is used to wage a political crusade against liberalism. This ideological shift represents a departure from traditional liberalism, seeking to establish a new modernity through the transformation of social structures of capitalist societies.

In the context of Fromm's theory, the concept of fascism is characterized by distinct features. This political form manifests characteristics that suggest a one-dimensional nature, exhibiting features reminiscent of authoritarianism. This phenomenon emerges from the sociopsychological conditions in which the masses organize themselves for national mobilization, driven by intense fear and loneliness. The rationale for its existence is contingent upon the power and influence of a charismatic leader.[79] Moreover, Fromm's conception of fascism as a form of authoritarianism suggests a pathological orientation and manner of governance characterized by "sadomasochism," a symbiotic relationship between sadism and masochism, in which sadistic and masochistic desires fuel a violent form of politics.[80] This perspective asserts that Fromm's subsequent literary works incorporated alternative character orientations, such as narcissism and necrophilia, into his theory of fascism. This integration occurred through the association of fascist politics with chauvinism and ethnonationalism; however, his landmark work, *Escape from Freedom*, primarily relied on the concept of the authoritarian personality to explain the origins of fascism.[81] This suggests that, in his later years, Fromm's research shifted toward examining the fascistic dynamics within the capitalist economy, which are rooted in narcissistic and necrophilous orientations.[82]

Fromm's conception of fascism is founded on a sociopsychological theoretical framework that utilizes Freudian psychoanalysis to elucidate socioeconomic structures. However, Fromm's focus on the modern concept of capitalism aligns with Griffin's perspective, suggesting a shared understanding that the capitalist economy serves as the underlying foundation of fascist politics. Nevertheless, it is argued that Fromm's conception of fascism holds a more pronounced theoretical relevance for today, particularly within the context of advanced countries. Fromm's concept of "pathological orientation and manner of governance" characterized by "sadomasochism" appears to be a more pertinent interpretation of contemporary political dynamics than Griffin's "revolutionary form of ultra-nationalism that attempts to realize the myth of the regenerated nation." It seems that none of the extant political systems that can be regarded as falling under the umbrella of fascism have undergone a revolutionary transformation in order to establish a nation that seeks the realization of "socio-political and cultural modernity," grounded in a particular nationalist ideology. Instead, it appears that these individuals are unconsciously engaged in sadomasochistic, symbiotic relationships, characterized by a focus on the gratification of narcissistic desires.[83] This is an accurate Frommian psychoanalytic sociotheoretical account of how the politics of fascist genealogy thrive in the current political climate.

In the context of US Trumpism, the concept of authoritarianism is noteworthy, and it can be posited that it manifests in a manner consistent with fascist ideology.[84] However, the authoritarian orientation does not appear to be a determining factor in the emergence of fascism in the contemporary political landscape. In this context, it may prove relevant to point out that Fromm's primary focus is on the role of narcissism in the development of fascist politics, as evidenced in his subsequent works, particularly in *The Heart of Man* (1964). In today's political landscape, narcissism has emerged as a critical component in the development of ideologies that fall under the umbrella of fascism. In my estimation, the overarching point about our politics is best understood by examining how authoritarian needs thrive in the context of political conditions rooted in narcissism, as opposed to merely assessing whether a social character exhibits an authoritarian orientation—it is evident that a comprehensive understanding of Fromm's social and political theories necessitates meticulous observation of *actual* political dynamics if their contemporary relevance is to be discerned. The character structure of narcissism is therefore enormously relevant to social and political theory, especially to theorizing about fascism—a topic that will be explored in greater detail in Chapter 4.

## Notes

1 Funk, *Das Leben selbst ist eine Kunst.*
2 Lesser, "Erich Fromm and the Psychoanalysis of the Social Unconscious."
3 Sakurai, *Political Theories of Narcissism*, 150.
4 W. Keith Campbell and Joshua D. Miller (Eds), *The Handbook of Narcissism and Narcissistic Personality Disorder: Theoretical Approaches, Empirical Findings, and Treatments* (Hoboken, NJ: John Wiley & Sons, 2011).
5 Elsa F. Ronningstam, *Identifying and Understanding the Narcissistic Personality* (New York: Oxford University Press, 2005).
6 Sakurai, *Political Theories of Narcissism*, 164.
7 Sakurai, *Political Theories of Narcissism*, 164, 165.
8 Sakurai, *Political Theories of Narcissism*, 217.
9 This is a point that the young Fromm articulated explicitly in his dispute with Wilhelm Reich.
10 Fromm, "Sozialpsychologischer Teil"; Fromm et al., "Zweite Abteilung. Erhebungen."
11 Fromm, *Escape from Freedom*, chs. 5 and 6.
12 Fromm, *Escape from Freedom*, 141.
13 Fromm, *Escape from Freedom*, 36.
14 Fromm, *Escape from Freedom*, 36–37.
15 Fromm, *The Anatomy of Human Destructiveness.*
16 Fromm, *The Anatomy of Human Destructiveness*, 325.
17 Fromm, *The Anatomy of Human Destructiveness*, 330–332.
18 Fromm, *The Anatomy of Human Destructiveness*, 332.
19 Fromm, *The Anatomy of Human Destructiveness*, 338.
20 Fromm, *The Anatomy of Human Destructiveness*, 339.
21 Fromm, *The Anatomy of Human Destructiveness*, 280–324.
22 Fromm, *Beyond the Chains of Illusion*, ch. 6; Erich Fromm, *Marx's Concept of Man* (London: Bloomsbury Academic, 2013 [1961]); Marx, *Economic and Philosophical Manuscripts*, 73–216; cf. Enzo Lio, "Alienation as a Central Concept in Marxist and Frommian Humanism," Presentation at a German-Italian Seminar about Die Marx Rezeption Erich Fromms, Bologna, 17–19 February 1989 (www

.frommgesellschaft.eu/images/pdf–Dateien/Lio_E_1989b.pdf); Sakurai, "The Socio-Psychological Base of Contemporary Fascism in the World of Liberal Democracy."; Sakurai, "A Frommian Perspective on the Socio-Psychological Structure of Post-Fascism in Liberal Democracies."

23 Marx, *Economic and Philosophical Manuscripts*; Marx, *Capital*, vol. 1: *A Critique of Political Economy.*

24 Marx, *Economic and Philosophical Manuscripts*, 88.

25 Fromm, *Man for Himself.*

26 Fromm, *Man for Himself*, 67, 81.

27 Fromm, *Man for Himself*, 73.

28 Fromm, *Man for Himself*, 72, 68.

29 Fromm, *To Have or To Be?.*

30 Erich Fromm, *On Being Human* (New York: Continuum, 2005 [1997]), pt. III; Fromm, *To Have or To Be?* chs. 3, 7; cf. Sakurai, *Political Theories of Narcissism*, 168.

31 Fromm, *To Have or To Be?* 57.

32 Fromm, *To Have or To Be?* 63.

33 Fromm, *To Have or To Be?* 23.

34 Fromm, *To Have or To Be?* 16.

35 Fromm, *Marx's Concept of Man*, 47–48.

36 Sakurai, "A Frommian Perspective on the Socio-Psychological Structure of Post-Fascism in Liberal Democracies," 180.

37 Lesser, "Erich Fromm and the Psychoanalysis of the Social Unconscious"; cf. Sakurai, *Political Theories of Narcissism*, 149.

38 Bacciagaluppi, "Fromm's View on Narcissism and the Self"; Marco Bacciagaluppi, *Paradigms in Psychoanalysis: An Integration* (New York: Columbia University Press, 2012); Marco Bacciagaluppi and Romano Biancoli, "Frommian Themes in a Case of Narcissistic Personality Disorder," *Contemporary Psychoanalysis*, 29, no. 3 (1993): 441–52; Leonidas K. Cheliotis, "Violence and Narcissism: A Frommian Perspective on Destructiveness under Authoritarianism," *Canadian Journal of Sociology*, 36, no. 4 (2012): 337–60; Rainer Funk, "Narzissmus und Gewalttätigkeit gegen Fremdes," in Internationale Erich-Fromm-Gesellschaft (Ed.), *Jahrbuch der Internationalen Erich-Fromm-Gesellschaft, vol. 5: Vom Umgang mit dem Fremden (Dealing with the Alien)* (Münster: LIT Verlag, 1993), 45–60; Rainer Funk, "Egoismus als Selbstsucht und Narzissmus: Überlegungen in Anschluss an Erich Fromm," in Thomas Leon Heck (Ed.), *Das Prinzip Egoismus* (Tübingen: Nous Verlag, 1994), 353–66; Rainer Funk, "The Continuing Relevance of Erich Fromm," *Fromm Forum* (English edn.), 4 (2000): 9–14; Kellner, "Donald Trump as Authoritarian Populist," 71–82; Sakurai, *Political Theories of Narcissism*; "The Socio-Psychological Base of Contemporary Fascism in the World of Liberal Democracy"; "A Frommian Perspective on the Socio-Psychological Structure of Post-Fascism in Liberal Democracies."

39 Bacciagaluppi, "Fromm's View on Narcissism and the Self," 93; cf. Sakurai, *Political Theories of Narcissism*; "The Socio-Psychological Base of Contemporary Fascism in the World of Liberal Democracy"; "A Frommian Perspective on the Socio-Psychological Structure of Post-Fascism in Liberal Democracies."

40 Freud, "On Narcissism: An Introduction," at 73–74.

41 Fromm, *The Art of Loving*; cf. Cheliotis, "Violence and Narcissism"; Sakurai, *Political Theories of Narcissism*; "The Socio-Psychological Base of Contemporary Fascism in the World of Liberal Democracy"; "A Frommian Perspective on the Socio-Psychological Structure of Post-Fascism in Liberal Democracies."

42 Erich Fromm, *The Sane Society* (New York: Henry Holt & Company, 1956 [1955]); Fromm, *The Art of Loving, Man for Himself.*

43 Fromm, *The Art of Loving*, 60–61; cf. Sakurai, *Political Theories of Narcissism*, 49–50.
44 Fromm, *Escape from Freedom*, 116; Fromm, *The Sane Society*, 36; Fromm, *The Art of Loving*, 60–61; Fromm, *Man for Himself*, 131.
45 Fromm, *Escape from Freedom*, 116.
46 Fromm, *The Anatomy of Human Destructiveness*, 201.
47 Fromm, *The Art of Loving*, 60.
48 Fromm, *The Heart of Man*, ch. 4.
49 Fromm, *The Heart of Man*, 77.
50 Fromm, *The Heart of Man*, 77.
51 Fromm, *The Heart of Man*, 72–73, 78; cf. Sakurai, *Political Theories of Narcissism*, 166.
52 Fromm, *The Heart of Man*, 78; cf. Sakurai, *Political Theories of Narcissism*, 51–54.
53 cf. Rainer Funk, "Fromm's Method of Social Psychology," Lecture at the American Academy of Psychoanalysis, 34th Winter Meeting, Hilton Palacio del Rio, San Antonio, Texas, US, 8 December 1990 (http://opus4.kobv.de/opus4Fromm/files /9899/Funk_R_1990e.pdf.1990).
54 Grey, "Society as Destiny."; cf. Sakurai, *Political Theories of Narcissism*, 158.
55 Erich Fromm, "The Method and Function of an Analytic Social Psychology: Notes on Psychoanalysis and Historical Materialism," in E. Fromm, *The Crisis of Psychoanalysis: Essays on Freud, Marx, and Social Psychology* (New York: Henry Holt & Company, 1970 [1932]), 135–162.
56 Fromm, *The Heart of Man*; Erich Fromm, *Greatness and Limitations of Freud's Thought* (London: Jonathan Cape, 1980 [1979]).
57 Fromm, *The Anatomy of Human Destructiveness*, 205.
58 Fromm, *The Anatomy of Human Destructiveness*, chs. 12 and 13.
59 Fromm, *The Heart of Man*, 78–79; cf. Sakurai, *Political Theories of Narcissism*, 51–52.
60 Fromm, *The Heart of Man*, 73–78.
61 Fromm, *The Heart of Man*, 85–87; cf. Sakurai, *Political Theories of Narcissism*, 52–53; Sakurai, "The Socio-Psychological Base of Contemporary Fascism in the World of Liberal Democracy," at 152.
62 Fromm, *The Heart of Man*, 80.
63 Fromm, *Greatness and Limitations of Freud's Thought*, 51–52; cf. Sakurai *Political Theories of Narcissism*, ch. 4, sect. 4.1.2; Thompson 2020, 39.
64 Fromm, *The Heart of Man*, 83; cf. Fromm, *The Anatomy of Human Destructiveness*, 300–1.
65 Fromm, *The Heart of Man*, 73.
66 Fromm, *The Heart of Man*, 86.
67 Fromm, *The Heart of Man*, 108–14.
68 See, e.g., Fromm, *The Heart of Man*, *The Anatomy of Human Destructiveness*.
69 Theodor W. Adorno and Max Horkheimer, *Dialectic of Enlightenment: Philosophical Fragments* (Stanford, CA: Stanford University Press, 2002).
70 Fromm, *Greatness and Limitations of Freud's* Thought, 53–54.
71 Fromm, *Greatness and Limitations of Freud's* Thought, 53–54.
72 Fromm, *The Heart of Man*, 87.
73 Sakurai, *Political Theories of Narcissism*, 53–56; Sakurai, "The Socio-Psychological Base of Contemporary Fascism in the World of Liberal Democracy," 152–53.
74 John Whittam, *Fascist Italy* (Manchester and New York: Manchester University Press, 1995), 6; cf. Sakurai, "The Socio-Psychological Base of Contemporary Fascism in the World of Liberal Democracy," 145.

75 Maurizio Bach, "Fascism," in Austin Harrington, Barbara L. Marshall, and Hans-Peter Muller (Eds), *Encyclopedia of Social Theory* (London and New York: Routledge, 2006), 192–93; Federico Finchelstein, *From Fascism to Populism in History* (Oakland, California: University of California Press, 2017); Roger Griffin, "Studying Fascism in a Postfascist Age: From New Consensus to New Wave?" *Fascism: Journal of Comparative Fascist Studies*, 1 (2012): 1–17; Kevin Passmore, *Fascism: A Very Short Introduction* (Oxford: Oxford University Press, 2014 [2002]); Whittam, *Fascist Italy*.
76 Bach, "Fascism," 192.
77 Griffin, "Studying Fascism in a Postfascist Age," 1.
78 Griffin, "Studying Fascism in a Postfascist Age," 1.
79 Fromm, *Escape from Freedom*; cf. Joan Braune, "Conclusion: Why Anti-Fascism Needs Erich Fromm's Critical Theory," in Joan Braune and Kieran Durkin (Eds), *Erich Fromm's Critical Theory: Hope, Humanism, and the Future* (London: Bloomsbury Academic, 2020), 216–26; McLaughlin, "Nazism, Nationalism, and the Sociology of Emotions"; Sakurai, "A Frommian Perspective on the Socio-Psychological Structure of Post-Fascism in Liberal Democracies."
80 Fromm, *Escape from Freedom*, chs. 5 and 6.
81 Fromm, *The Heart of Man*, *The Anatomy of Human Destructiveness*, *To Have or To Be?*
82 Fromm, *The Heart of Man*, *To Have or To Be?*
83 Kellner, "Donald Trump as Authoritarian Populist"; Sakurai, "A Frommian Perspective on the Socio-Psychological Structure of Post-Fascism in Liberal Democracies"; cf. Enzo Traverso, *The New Faces of Fascism: Populism and the Far Right*, David Broder (Trans.) (London: Verso, 2019).
84 See, e.g., Carl Boggs, *Fascism Old and New: American Politics at the Crossroads* (Abingdon, Oxon: Routledge, 2018); William E. Connolly, *Aspirational Fascism: The Struggle for Multifaceted Democracy under Trumpism* (Minneapolis: University of Minnesota Press, 2017); Henry A. Giroux, *American Nightmare: Facing the Challenge of Fascism* (San Francisco: City Lights Books, 2018); Jason Stanley, *How Fascism Works: The Politics of US and Them* (New York: Random House, 2018).

# 3 Perception of Fromm in Political Theory

## Reception History of Fromm

Fromm's contributions have been predominantly recognized within the fields of philosophy, sociology, and psychoanalysis. This recognition appears to be the consequence of his academic endeavors, which were predominantly focused on these disciplines. Despite the transdisciplinary nature of his oeuvre, Fromm has not received sufficient attention from politics and political theory that he merits—this issue is likewise regarded in a similar vein to the precise stipulation of disregarding his psychoanalytic compositions, as previously observed. A distinguishing feature of this oversight is the tendency to overshadow Fromm's political thought within the broader context of his sociological and sociotheoretical contributions. As a result, political theory has historically overlooked him within the purview of theoretical disciplines.

Nevertheless, it seems likely that the apparent oversight in the field of political theory is partly due to the fragmentation of academic disciplines—thus, the oversight is not primarily attributable to this environmental factor. A comprehensive evaluation of Fromm's body of work reveals a marked deviation from established academic conventions. This deviation can be ascribed mainly to the reluctance of prominent academic figures to acknowledge the merits of his work. This observation unveils a salient fact: Fromm's marginal position was primarily influenced by the prevailing intellectual discourse among prominent scholars in academic fields.

From this perspective, it can be posited that Fromm's academic contributions have been deliberately overlooked or circumvented, rather than being disregarded or disdained in the literal sense of the word. If the hypothesis that the compartmentalization of disciplines is the primary factor in his disregard is accurate, then other scholars who similarly engaged in interdisciplinary work around the early and mid-twentieth century should face a similar fate. A comprehensive overview of this phenomenon can be achieved through a comparative analysis of Fromm with other prominent figures of his generation who were affiliated with the Frankfurt Institute for Social Research. While it is challenging to identify another scholar who operated at the same interdisciplinary level as Fromm, notable figures such as Herbert Marcuse

DOI: 10.4324/9781003600398-4

(1898–1979) and Walter Benjamin (1892–1940) are particularly pertinent in this context. A notable point of convergence between the two scholars is their shared birthplace, Germany, as well as their shared status as scholars in Fromm's generation. A salient point of comparison is Marcuse's emigration to the United States during a period analogous to that of Fromm's, thereby underscoring the transnational and comparative dimensions of their intellectual and academic trajectories.

Marcuse was born in Berlin approximately two years prior to Fromm's birth in the late nineteenth century. A notable point of interest is the synchrony of Marcuse's emigration to the United States in 1934, which occurred in the same year as Fromm's relocation to the same country. Marcuse's areas of expertise encompass philosophy, social theory, sociology, and psychoanalysis. Among the various critical theorists, Marcuse's proximity to Fromm is particularly notable. Marcuse initiated his academic inquiry into Hegel's philosophy under the mentorship of Husserl and Heidegger. Marcuse is perhaps most renowned for his 1964 work *One-Dimensional Man*, which provides a penetrating analysis of both capitalist and communist societies in the mid-twentieth century. Another noteworthy work is *Eros and Civilization* (1955), a previous publication by him, which draws upon Freud's theory of instinct and proposes a repressive model of society, along with a corresponding remedy.

During his active period, Marcuse had already achieved renown as a scholarly figure and had received particular acclaim from radical leftists.[1] His thought proved particularly appealing to young students engaged in radical activism, and it received significant media attention, leading to his portrayal as the "Father of the New Left."[2]

It is plausible to regard Benjamin as a distinctive figure among critical theorists. He was born almost eight years earlier than Fromm's birth. While Benjamin's early academic endeavors were concentrated in philosophy, his intellectual curiosity transcended traditional boundaries, encompassing a diverse array of disciplines, including aesthetics, literary theory, philosophy of history, poetry, and even theology. This intellectual breadth is exemplified by his seminal work, *Theses on the Philosophy of History*, written in the early 1940s. Guided by his personal existentialist perspective, Benjamin cultivated a profound interest in Judaism, though he refrained from overt political engagement. Instead, he aligned himself with a variant of Zionism he termed "cultural Zionism," emphasizing its cultural and ideological aspects.[3] Notwithstanding his evident intellectual aptitude, Benjamin encountered significant challenges in his academic career, a trajectory that stands in stark contrast to the trajectory of Marcuse, as previously observed. In a moment of profound desperation, Benjamin took his own life in Portbou, Catalonia, while attempting to evade the Nazi regime. Prior to this incident, Benjamin procured a travel visa for the United States from Max Horkheimer.

Although only a minority may consider Benjamin's contributions to be interdisciplinary in a Frommian sense, it is evident that his influence extends to a diverse array of disciplines, including, but not limited to, aesthetics, history, literary theory, philosophy, poetry, political theory, social theory, and theology. In the contemporary academic landscape, Benjamin's contributions to critical theory have been the subject of extensive debate and scrutiny. It is imperative to acknowledge, however, that his oeuvre has already garnered significant acclaim and recognition during the twentieth century.[4]

In light of the aforementioned brief survey, the apparent difficulty in comprehending Fromm's interdisciplinary approach is not, in fact, an impediment. The underlying reason for this oversight appears to be a *deliberate disregard*. The period under discussion was distinguished by a remarkable prevalence of interdisciplinary scholars, a phenomenon that far exceeded contemporary standards. This assertion finds notable application in the context of critical theorists. Even in contemporary society, there is a discernible appreciation for figures who operate within a highly interdisciplinary framework, particularly within the ambit of critical theory. Jürgen Habermas is a prominent exemplar of this phenomenon and is undoubtedly the most respected critical theorist today. While his primary field of study is philosophy, his areas of expertise are extensive and include highly specialized disciplines such as law. His reception appears to be largely influenced by the very interdisciplinarity of his academic pursuits. From this perspective, the interdisciplinary nature of critical theory is precisely an attractive quality for the target audience.

In essence, *preferences* function as the predominant determinants of evaluation. As Fromm himself asserts, one's value is determined by whether one is liked by others.[5] Fromm's assertion that the twentieth century was characterized by this approach is not accurate; it appears that the twenty-first century is more characterized by it. This observation indicates that human existence, particularly within the paradigm of market society, is significantly influenced by this evaluation system, or more precisely, the evaluation *habit*—it seems that the evaluation scale of preferences is compatible with authoritarianism. However, this phenomenon is not exclusive to the capitalist market but is also evident in academic settings. In contemporary academic society, the extent to which one's professional accomplishments and professional demeanor are evaluated by a substantial number of prominent academic figures serves as the prevailing and most potent evaluation system—this phenomenon underscores the authoritarian nature of academia. To summarize, a significant majority of the academics displayed *a lack of interest* in Fromm's oeuvre, and some even expressed *disfavor* toward it.

It is evident that academic disregard does not serve as a determining factor in an individual's academic value. This assertion is particularly salient in the context of contemporary critics who advocate for free thought. Indeed, Fromm has garnered appraisals from external sources, largely from beyond the confines of academic circles.[6] However, this phenomenon is not confined to the period of Fromm; rather, it is highly relevant to the present period. In the contemporary academic landscape, marked by its extensive institutionalization, the prospect of independent scholarly pursuits has become increasingly constrained. Therefore, it can be argued that individuals harboring idiosyncratic intellectual concepts may find it more feasible to articulate these from a marginal vantage point. This assertion highlights the significance of a considerable degree of autonomy, or a substantial distance, from the prevailing academic milieu for individuals who possess unconventional intellectual concepts. I believe that Fromm was among their number and was acutely aware of this vexing fact.

Notwithstanding the aforementioned fact, Fromm has gained recognition for his interdisciplinary approach in recent years, as mentioned in the Introduction. Fromm's "sociopsychoanalytic approach" has recently garnered significant acclaim, particularly following the reaffirmation of the objective of his theory to "integrate psychoanalysis and sociology." However, a substantial portion of the discourse does not constitute a continuation of Fromm's critical theory in its strictest sense. Most individuals primarily focus on the interpretation, analysis, and clinical application of Fromm's theoretical framework—it appears that their primary objective does not encompass the advancement of his theoretical concepts or the societal transformation (enhancement) they might engender.

Despite the aforementioned critical appraisal of Fromm, I maintain its pertinence, particularly within the realm of social theory. This assertion is founded on the premise that social theory constitutes the primary theoretical function of critical theory. Moreover, Fromm's theoretical framework is most appropriately characterized as critical theory. Of course, reception from disparate fields can be discernible and pertinent nowadays. Fromm's philosophical oeuvre, inclusive of his social theory, has received considerable acclaim within relevant academic circles.[7] Despite the pervasive lack of recognition of Fromm in the mainstream of the field, psychoanalysis has made a substantial contribution to Fromm studies.[8] The academic field of sociology has demonstrated a favorable reception of Fromm's contributions, exhibiting a congruence in its response with that observed in psychoanalysis.[9] Psychology has contributed to Fromm studies in several ways. A comparative analysis reveals that, in contrast to the significant influence of these disciplines, the impact of political theory on Fromm research has been comparatively negligible. Nonetheless, critical theory has contributed to the development of Fromm's work within the discipline of political theory. This, it is argued, has exerted a favorable influence on Fromm research, particularly in the sense that Fromm is best construed as a critical theorist.

A review of the extant literature reveals a conspicuous absence of attention to the contributions of Fromm in the field of political theory. As previously stated, this phenomenon appears to be closely associated with Fromm's academic endeavors per se, albeit to a lesser extent with regard to political science and political theory. In the following sections, I undertake a rigorous examination of the fundamental concepts that Fromm investigated in relation to the framework of disciplinary approaches in political theory, with a particular focus on authoritarianism, fascism, and alienation. The primary inquiry concerns the manner in which Fromm's theoretical contributions have been referenced within the context of these three themes, and the manner in which the principles of political theory have been intertwined with his theoretical contributions.

### Authoritarianism

The term "authoritarianism" is currently employed to denote authoritarian regimes, with its usage being exclusively associated with the realm of politics. Conversely, the concept of the "authoritarian personality" appears to be predominantly utilized in a standalone manner within the realm of psychology.[10] The discourse on this subject within these disciplines is characterized by its marked degree of specialization, which can pose a substantial challenge for individuals lacking specialized knowledge in the field. The primary objective of this section is to decipher the transformation of the concept of the authoritarian personality from a sociopsychological theoretical construct to a psychological construct that is empirically substantiated, as well as the transformation of the concept of authoritarianism from it into a politically empirical construct.

In the field of political science, authoritarianism is defined as a political system characterized by a strong central government, where power is concentrated in the hands of a select few. The concept of "competitive authoritarianism" has been employed to delineate a particular manifestation of authoritarianism, one that is typified by the existence of a competitive electoral system, a hallmark of the present-day political landscape. It is indicative of specific political systems of governance in a limited sense within the discipline of political science, particularly in the context of comparative politics. Conversely, the authoritarian personality is characterized by a conventional emphasis on the psychological and sociopsychological dimensions of authoritarian figures and groups. The significance of this concept lies in its role in personality, disposition, and attitude. The concept under scrutiny encompasses the psychologies of the individual and society as a whole, along with their various forms. A compelling illustration of the distinction between authoritarianism and the authoritarian personality can be observed in the case of Donald Trump and his administration. Within the theoretical framework of competitive authoritarianism, the Trump government does not inherently embody authoritarian tendencies; however, it does exhibit characteristics of authoritarianism in terms of the authoritarian personality. This suggests that the latter is intended to refer to the concepts of authoritarian figure "Trump" and authoritarian politics "Trumpism," irrespective of whether or not scholars are cognizant of this signification.

During the early twentieth century, the term "authoritarianism" had not yet been adopted as an academic concept. The concept of the authoritarian personality is derived from the early Frankfurt School's project *Studien über Autorität und Familie* (Studies on Authority and Family) (1936), particularly Fromm's theoretical contribution.[11] This phenomenon constitutes the theoretical foundation of the concept of authoritarianism. However, the concept was incorporated into the field of psychology through Adorno's empirical research conducted in conjunction with psychologists around 1950.[12] Subsequent to that period, the term has been utilized exclusively within the domain of psychology, encompassing various empirical subfields, including social psychology. Similarly, the concept of authoritarianism came to the fore as a distinct empirical framework within the realm of political science during the 1960s. The political scientist Juan Linz theorized it as an empirically based political concept in his pioneering work *An Authoritarian Regime: Spain* (1964), which employs an academic lens to characterize the Francoist regime in Spain as an authoritarian system.[13] In the twenty-first century, Steven Levitsky and Lucan A. Way refined the concept of authoritarianism in a more appropriate fashion after Cold War political regimes in their 2010 publication, *Competitive Authoritarianism: Hybrid Regimes after the Cold War*.[14]

As a result, the concept of authoritarianism has been distinctly disassociated from that of the authoritarian personality. The former has been exclusively an empirically oriented political concept, while the latter has been exclusively an empirically oriented psychological concept. Contemporary political scientists employ the term "authoritarianism" exclusively in a Linzian sense, while psychologists, including social and political psychologists, utilize the concept of the "authoritarian personality" solely within the realm of psychology, disregarding its essential political connotation. In Fromm's conception, authoritarianism is synonymous with the authoritarian personality, and vice versa. As has been demonstrated above, the notion of authoritarianism is derived from the concept of the authoritarian personality. However, the extant evidence does not provide robust support for a direct correlation between the two. This observation suggests the presence of a considerable degree of irony.

The extant evidence suggests the presence of two distinct interpretations of the concept of authoritarianism, each of which is utilized in different academic realms, namely political science and psychology. Critical theory employs the concept almost exclusively in the sense of the authoritarian personality.[15] Within the framework of academic classification, philosophy, social theory, and political theory use the concept in a manner consistent with critical theory.[16] The term "authoritarianism," as employed in a Linzian sense, is exclusively utilized within the domain of empirical political science. In contrast, the term "authoritarian personality" appears to be more extensively applied beyond the confines of political science, as mentioned previously. This survey posits that the application of authoritarianism, in the sense of the authoritarian personality, is predominantly used within the paradigm of critical theory.

In the context of Fromm's theoretical framework, authoritarianism is conceptualized as exclusively denoting the authoritarian personality. This observation clearly demonstrates that contemporary empirical political science does not engage with Fromm's theory of authoritarianism. As previously indicated, this book puts forth the hypothesis that, given the connotations of the notion, the concept in question primarily pertains to the authoritarian personality in the context of the humanities and social sciences. This assertion is substantiated by the extensive referencing of Fromm in these disciplines, thereby underscoring the relevance of his theoretical contributions to these academic fields.

In the English-language context, the predominant tendency to cite Fromm's theory of authoritarianism has been observed within the domains of critical theory, encompassing philosophy, social theory, and sociology,[17] as well as clinical and behavioral disciplines, comprising psychoanalysis, psychology, and psychiatry.[18] As anticipated, references to Fromm in political theory are rather limited, while empirical political science contains a specific number of references to him, yet exclusively in relation to the authoritarian personality theory.[19] This phenomenon can be attributed, at least in part, to the academic disciplines in which Fromm primarily engaged, as previously indicated. In the context of the authoritarian personality theory, it is noteworthy that the names "Fromm" and "Adorno" are frequently cited in conjunction.[20] Within the domain of psychology, the latter appellation is predominant, particularly in academic discourse.[21] This phenomenon appears to stem from two factors. First, there is a lack of direct concern for Fromm within the theoretical framework. Second, there is a paucity of knowledge regarding the theoretical underpinnings of the theory. Conversely, a number of scholars in the humanities, including those specializing in philosophy and social theory, have exhibited a direct interest in Fromm's theories regarding the concept of authoritarianism. However, these scholars appear to rarely mention Fromm's theory of authoritarianism in isolation; rather, they tend to discuss it within the broader context of his critical social theory. In this regard, the contributions of Fromm must be considered more central than is often the case with the authoritarian personality theory. For instance, Douglas Kellner (2016) alludes to Fromm in the context of his comprehensive social theory.[22] Kellner's analysis encompasses not only Fromm's theory of authoritarianism but also his other theories of narcissism, necrophilia, and aggression, which intersect with the former. Kellner employs a Frommian lens to examine Trumpism in its broader context. Cristian Fuchs (2018) situates Fromm's authoritarianism within a broader discourse encompassing fascism and capitalism.[23] Despite the limited scope of Fuchs's reference, his interest in Fromm is evident. Significant contributions to Fromm's thought can be identified in the disciplines of social theory and sociology, particularly with regard to authoritarianism.[24]

Despite the challenges in identifying books on Fromm's theory of authoritarianism (or more accurately, the authoritarian personality) in clinical fields, such as psychoanalysis and psychiatry, a substantial corpus of articles that refer to this theory exists within these disciplines.[25] In the context of psychiatric and psychoanalytic discourse, the theory is predominantly constrained to the individual level—this limitation is inherent to the nature of the subjects under scrutiny by these disciplines.

A substantial corpus of literature has been published in the field of psychology, yet only a limited number of works make extensive reference to Fromm's theory of authoritarianism. *Political Psychology: Key Readings* (2004), a collection edited by John Jost and Jim Sidanius, dedicates a section to the authoritarian personality, drawing upon the theoretical contributions of Fromm.[26] *An Introduction to Theories of Personality,* 7th Edition (2010), edited by Robert E. Ewen, contains a contribution to Fromm's psychological theory.[27] These works are more specific to psychology than to politics and extensively focus on personality theory. It is therefore conceivable that the phenomena delineated in these texts have been overlooked by philosophers and social theorists. It is noteworthy that the authors draw attention to Fromm's sociopsychological theory in its totality.

Conversely, it is challenging to identify works on Fromm in the domain of political theory. In the academic literature, David Spitz's *Democracy and the Challenge of Power* (1958), Christian Bay's *The Structure of Freedom* (1965), and A. James Gregor's *Fascism* (1973) all make reference to Fromm's theory of authoritarianism. However, the role of Fromm is only mentioned in passing in these texts. The political theorist Stephen Eric Bronner is distinctive in this field. His literary contributions, including the Oxford series of *Very Short Introductions*, *Critical Theory* (2011), and *Of Critical Theory and Its Theorists* (1994), are regarded as significant contributions to the field of political theory. A comprehensive review of both books reveals a substantial use of references to Fromm, albeit with a restriction to his theory of authoritarianism. The focus of the texts does not extend beyond this theoretical framework. Nevertheless, the primary focus of this book is the political aspects of authoritarianism, with a particular emphasis on its semantic implications concerning the authoritarian personality. It is noteworthy to cite Lawrence Wilde's *Erich Fromm and the Quest for Solidarity* (2004), which undertakes an examination of Fromm's conception of authoritarianism.[28] This work stands as a singular English-language book on Fromm within the contemporary state of this field, with the exception of the present book.

It is notable that Bronner's and Wilde's works are particularly noteworthy in their employment of Fromm's concept of authoritarianism, which is situated within the broader framework of his theory of social character. The commonalities between political theory and other humanities fields, such as philosophy and social theory, have become a subject of significant scholarly interest. In essence, their primary concern is to discern authoritarian elements within society by employing authoritarianism as a conceptual framework, thereby identifying antidemocratic orientations within democratic societies. This perspective finds close alignment with Fromm's theoretical framework of authoritarianism, a conceptual model developed to elucidate the dynamics of authoritarian orientations.

## Fascism

Fascism is a fundamental political concept in Fromm's theoretical framework. This is due to the fact that Fromm's primary objective in conducting his academic research was to combat fascist politics. In fact, his magnum opus, *Escape from Freedom*, is a direct exposition of this struggle. A salient aspect of his theory of fascism is its theoretical foundation in authoritarianism. This finding suggests that the concept draws considerable inspiration from his other theory of authoritarianism. Moreover, sadomasochism is predicated on Fromm's authoritarian theory, as expounded in the preceding chapter, thereby rendering his theory of fascism more intricate.

While critical theory has undoubtedly contributed significantly to the field of Fromm research in this area, it does not represent the majority of contributions. Moreover, this theme does not restrict scholars to the traditionally predominant fields concerning Fromm's theory, such as philosophy, psychoanalysis, and social theory. A variety of academic disciplines have approached Fromm's theory of fascism, including history, literature, political science, political theory, psychology, and sociology, in addition to the previously noted disciplines. In the English-language context, notable contributions from critical theory include Christian Fuchs's *Digital Fascism* (2022), Joan Braune's *Understanding and Countering Fascist Movements* (2023), Geoff M. Boucher's *Critical Theory and the Authoritarian Personality* (2025), and Jeremiah Morelock's *Critical Theory and Authoritarian Populism* (2018) and *How to Critique Authoritarian Populism* (2021).[29] As indicated by the titles of these works, their focus does not pertain to Fromm; however, they do make extensive references to his theory.

With regard to the subject of fascism, the most prominent figure is indisputably the political theorist Roger Griffin. *The Nature of Fascism* (1991) is a foundational work on the subject. Griffin defines fascism as a "revolutionary form of ultra-nationalism that attempts to realize the myth of the regenerated nation."[30] He argues that fascism functions as an alternative to "liberal capitalism" and a nationalist ideology that is utilized to initiate a political crusade against liberalism.[31] Griffin's analysis draws, in some part, on the work of Fromm, particularly in the context of fascist ideologies.[32] Another noteworthy work in the realm of political theory is James Gregor's *Interpretations of Fascism* (2017).[33] In this book, Gregor's concern is with the authoritarian personality, which Fromm articulates in *Escape from Freedom*. In alignment with the central theme of *Escape from Freedom*, Jon Delogu's *Fascism, Vulnerability, and Escape from Freedom* (2022) emerges as a noteworthy publication.[34] In this book, Delogu engages with Fromm's magnum opus in a dedicated chapter, offering a comprehensive analysis of its extensive content.

Historical approaches are also worth noting. Walter Laqueur's *Fascism* (1976) employs an interpretive framework informed by Fromm's theories, contextualizing historical fascism within a sociopsychological interpretation.[35] In Martin Kitchen's *Fascism* (1976), Fromm's *Escape from Freedom* is cited as a seminal work, underscoring its significance in the field.[36] Avihu Zakai's *Jewish Exiles' Psychological Interpretations of Nazism* (2020) makes extensive reference to Fromm, aligning him with other German Jewish scholars of his generation.[37]

Notably, the field of psychology also contributes to Fromm research in this area. Israel Charny's *Fascism and Democracy in the Human Mind* (2006) is a seminal sociopsychological work, as the Israeli author tackles the issues of the Holocaust.[38] In this work, Charny references *Escape from Freedom* in the dialectic of fascism and democracy in the hope that the latter fundamentally overcomes its own political contradiction, fascism. Additionally, Antonios Vadolas's *Perversions of Fascism* (2009) is a noteworthy reference work in this area.[39] With respect to Fromm, this book places particular emphasis on his formulation of a sociopsychological theory grounded in Freudian–Marxist tenets with the objective of elucidating the pernicious nature of fascist ideology. In Babak Fozooni's *Psychology, Humour and Class* (2020), significant attention is devoted to the examination of Fromm's contributions within a comprehensive sociopsychological framework, encompassing the subjects of political fascism, Freudian psychoanalysis, and sadomasochism.[40] In his recent book *Edge of Catastrophe* (2024), Roger Frie primarily examines Fromm's theory of fascism in terms of the Holocaust.[41] In the sense that the book is about Fromm's sociopsychological theory of fascism, it is worthwhile to reference it here. Yet, the most salient point is that it addresses racial correspondence in Fromm's family in the context of the Holocaust.

Sociology has also made significant remarks on Fromm's theory of fascism. Neil McLaughlin's work is characterized by a concerted effort to explore the potential of global public sociology through the lens of Fromm's theories.[42] Leighton Grist focuses on an examination of fascist orientations that have emerged within the context of American cinema.[43] A commonality among these works is their engagement with one of Fromm's seminal themes, fascism.

While a variety of themes are discernible in scholarly contributions to the subject of fascism in Fromm research, the central pillar is Fromm's conception of authoritarianism described in *Escape from Freedom*. A salient point of reference to Fromm is that referencing Fromm is to end up with his Freudian sociopsychological approach, even in the context of fascism. This observation suggests that Fromm's conception of fascism is comprised of his other theories of authoritarianism and sadomasochism, and that any discussion of Fromm's theory of fascism must necessarily encompass the latter two theories. This perspective explains why Fromm's conception of fascism is distinctive and interdisciplinarily compelling.

**Alienation**

The term "alienation" is a Marxist sociopathological concept that originated in Marx's philosophy. As I previously stated in Chapter 2, Fromm's primary source for this concept and its theoretical significance is Marx. In Fromm's social theory, this phenomenon functions as a significant catalyst for detrimental societal outcomes. With respect to alienation, it is noteworthy to refer particularly to his sociocharacterological theories of the marketing orientation and the having mode—for a detailed discussion of these concepts, see Chapter 2.

In the context of market capitalism, contemporary individuals prioritize the satisfaction of their personal needs through the pursuit of material possessions (having mode), while simultaneously aligning with societal expectations through a marketing-oriented approach (marketing orientation). This duality in approach is indicative of an attempt to respond to the demands of both individual and collective needs. Individuals therefore reinforce a sociocharacter structure that fosters alienation and compels them to adopt a passive role within the framework of market capitalism. In Fromm's perspective, alienation is perpetuated and its social condition is regenerated by both society and the individual. This dynamic enables both parties to achieve their respective objectives, with the latter adapting to the former and internalizing its needs, irrespective of social class. In this regard, individuals manifest self-destructive tendencies, stemming from their passive position under the influence of alienation, as conceptualized within Fromm's theoretical framework.

Research on this theme concerning Fromm's theory is also discernible in various fields, including literature, philosophy, political science, political theory, psychology, sociology, theology, and criminology. Yet, the field of philosophy most enthusiastically engages in the issues of alienation. Richard Schacht tackles them and cites Fromm's work extensively in his book, *Alienation* (1970), where Fromm is central to Schacht's discussion.[44] Christoph Henning (2024) also draws attention to some of the central themes on alienation, using the psychological concept of "estrangement" and referring to Fromm.[45] Psychology also contributes to this theme. Christopher J. Hewer's and Evanthia Lyons's *Political Psychology* (2018) puts space for Fromm in the theme of alienation.[46] Terry D. Cooper's *Paul Tillich and Psychology* (2006) references Fromm's theory of alienation to illuminate the theologian Paul Tillich's psychology.[47] Some of the other fields, such as policy studies, also reference Fromm. For example, Lars Tummers's *Policy Alienation and the Power of Professionals* (2013) introduces Fromm's theory of alienation for public management.[48] James A. Tyner's *The Alienated Subject* (2022) proposes the image of alienated individuals under twenty-first-century racial capitalism, referring to various thinkers including Fromm.[49] The edited book *Theories of Alienation* (1976) references Fromm, approaching alienation cross-disciplinarily from social philosophy to empirical social research.[50]

While direct contributions to Fromm research in this subject are certainly recognizable, the majority are confined to the research-paper level.[51] A seminal contribution to this subject is arguably *Erich Fromm and Critical Criminology*, edited by Kevin Anderson and Richard Quinney (2000), which examines alienation as a pivotal issue.[52] Lawrence Friedman's *The Lives of Erich Fromm* (2013) addresses Fromm's conception of alienation, but its issues are at the biographical level.[53]

It is evident that the direct contribution of political theory to this theme is not immediately apparent. However, Lawrence Wilde's *Erich Fromm and the Quest for Solidarity* (2004) addresses Fromm's issues of alienation, thereby suggesting a way out of them to achieve radical humanism. In this context, it is also pertinent to make reference to the author's book (2018).[54]

Despite the abundance of references to Fromm's alienation, there is a paucity of scholarship on the subject, particularly within the field of political theory. The majority of publications on this theme are composed of articles and research papers in cross-disciplinary fields, including philosophy, social theory, and psychoanalysis.[55] Moreover, research concerning Fromm's theory of alienation is predominantly characterized by a sociopathological orientation. This may be the reason why there has been minimal engagement with this subject in the realm of political theory.

## Notes

1 Herbert Marcuse, *From the New Left to the Next Left* (Lawrence, KS: University Press of Kansas, 1994).
2 Steven Loyal and Sinisa Malesevic, *Contemporary Sociological Theory* (London: Sage, 2020), 159.
3 Howard Eiland and Michael William Jennings, *Walter Benjamin: A Critical Life* (Cambridge, MA: Harvard University Press, 2014), 47; Anson Rabinbach, "Between Apocalypse and Enlightenment: Benjamin, Bloch and Modern German Jewish Messianism," in Peter Osborne (Ed.), *Walter Benjamin: Critical Evaluations in Cultural Theory*, Vol. 3 (Abingdon, Oxon: Routledge, 2005), 116–61, at 128.
4 Eiland and Jennings, *Walter Benjamin*.
5 Fromm, *Man for Himself*, 68–72.
6 See, e.g., David Ingleby, "Introduction to the Second Edition of *The Same Society*," in Erich Fromm, *The Sane Society* (Abingdon, Oxon: Routledge: 2002 [1955]), xvi–lv, at li.
7 See the Introduction.
8 Sakurai, *Political Theories of Narcissism*, ch. 6.
9 Takamichi Sakurai, "The Socio-Theoretical Relevance of Erich Fromm's Psychoanalytic Conception of Narcissism: Towards a Frommian Critical Social Theory of Narcissism," *Theoria*, 68, no. 1 (2021): 1–30, at 2.
10 Klaus Boehnke and Andreas Hadjar, "Authoritarianism," in Charles Spielberger (Ed.), *Encyclopedia of Applied Psychology*, Vol. 1 (Oxford, Boston: Elsevier Academic Press, 2004), 151–56.
11 Institut für Sozialforschung (Ed.), *Studien über Autorität und Familie*; Fromm, "Sozialpsychologischer Teil"; Fromm et al., "Zweite Abteilung. Erhebungen."
12 Theodor W. Adorno, Else Frenkel-Brunswik, Daniel J. Levinson, and R. Nevitt Sanford, *The Authoritarian Personality* (New York: Harper & Row, 1950).

13 Juan J. Linz, "An Authoritarian Regime: The Case of Spain," in Erik Allardt and Yrjö Littunen (Eds), *Cleavages, Ideologies, and Party Systems: Contributions to Comparative Political Sociology* (Helsinki: Academic Bookstore, 1964), 291–341.

14 Steven Levitsky and Lucan A. Way, *Competitive Authoritarianism: Hybrid Regimes after the Cold War* (New York: Cambridge University Press, 2010).

15 Wendy Brown, Peter E. Gordon, and Max Pensky, *Authoritarianism: Three Inquiries in Critical Theory* (Chicago: University of Chicago Press, 2018); Christian Fuchs, *Digital Demagogue: Authoritarian Capitalism in the Age of Trump and Twitter* (London: Pluto Press, 2018); Kellner, *American Nightmare*; Jeremiah Morelock (Ed.), *Critical Theory and Authoritarian Populism* (London: University of Westminster Press, 2018).

16 In addition to the publications in note 15 above, consult the following sources limited to Fromm research: Joan Braune, *Understanding and Countering Fascist Movements: From Void to Hope* (Abingdon, Oxon: Routledge, 2023); Braune and Durkin (Eds), *Erich Fromm's Critical Theory*; Joseph Fantauzzi, Maor Levitin, and Terry Maley (Eds), *Erich Fromm and Left Strategy: New Paths Toward Radical Transformation* (Cham, Switzerland: Palgrave Macmillan, 2025); Takamichi Sakurai, "The Authoritarian Orientation in Liberal Democracies: Labor Market and Workplace Authoritarianism," *Constellations* 32, no. 1 (2015): 59–68.

17 See, e.g., Braune, *Understanding and Countering Fascist Movements*; Braune and Durkin, *Erich Fromm's Critical Theory*; Fuchs, *Digital Demagogue*; Kellner, *American Nightmare*; Morelock, *Critical Theory and Authoritarian Populism.*

18 See, e.g., Bob Altemeyer, "The Other Authoritarian Personality," in John T. Jost and Jim Sidanius (Eds), *Political Psychology: Key Readings* (New York: Psychology Press, 2004), 85–107; Boehnke and Hadjar, "Authoritarianism"; Mauricio Cortina, "Prologue: Erich Fromm's Relevance for Our Troubled World," *Psychoanalytic Inquiry* 44, no. 1 (2024): 1–8; Else Frenkel-Brunswik and *The Authoritarian Personality*," in Vlad Petre Glaveanu (Ed.), *The Creativity Reader* (New York: Oxford University Press, 2019), 517–32; Roger Frie, *Edge of Catastrophe: Erich Fromm, Fascism, and the Holocaust* (New York: Oxford University Press, 2024); Peter L. Rudnytsky, "The Social Determinants of Psychoanalytic Therapy: Fromm's Anti-Authoritarian 'Calling Card,'" *Psychoanalytic Inquiry* 44, no. 1 (2024): 9–14.

19 Peter Merrotsy, "Authoritarian Personality," in Fathali M. Moghaddam (Ed.), *The SAGE Encyclopedia of Political Behavior* (London: Sage, 2017), 45–47; Pippa Norris and Ronald Inglehart, *Cultural Backlash: Trump, Brexit, and Authoritarian Populism* (Cambridge: Cambridge University Press, 2019).

20 See, e.g., George Lundskow, *The Sociology of Religion: A Substantive and Transdisciplinary Approach* (London: Sage, 2008), 37; Judd Marmor, *Modern Psychoanalysis: New Directions and Perspectives* (New York: Basic Books, 1968), 609; Carter A. Wilson, *Trumpism: Race, Class, Populism, and Public Policy* (Lexington, MA: Lexington Books, 2021), 27.

21 Altemeyer, "The Other Authoritarian Personality"; Boehnke and Hadjar, "Authoritarianism"; Montuori, "Authoritarianism and Creativity."

22 See note 15.

23 See note 15.

24 Braune and Durkin, *Erich Fromm's Critical Theory*; Morelock, *Critical Theory and Authoritarian Populism.*

25 See, e.g., Cortina, "Prologue: Erich Fromm's Relevance for Our Troubled World"; Rudnytsky, "The Social Determinants of Psychoanalytic Therapy."

26 See note 18.

27 Robert B. Ewen, *An Introduction to Theories of Personality,* 7th ed. (New York: Psychology Press, 2014).

28 Wilde, *Erich Fromm and the Quest for Solidarity.*
29 Braune, *Understanding and Countering Fascist Movements*; Geoff M. Boucher, *Critical Theory and the Authoritarian Personality* (Edinburgh: Edinburgh University Press, 2025); Christian Fuchs, *Digital Fascism: Media, Communication and Society Volume Four* (Abingdon, Oxon: Routledge, 2022); Morelock, *Critical Theory and Authoritarian Populism*; Jeremiah Morelock (Ed.), *How to Critique Authoritarian Populism: Methodologies of the Frankfurt School* (Leiden and Boston: Brill, 2021).
30 Griffin, "Studying Fascism in a Postfascist Age, " at 1.
31 Griffin, "Studying Fascism in a Postfascist Age."
32 Roger Griffin, *A Fascist Century: Essays by Roger Griffin* (Houndmills, Basingstoke, Hampshire: Palgrave Macmillan, 2008).
33 A. James Gregor, *Interpretations of Fascism* (Abingdon, Oxon: Routledge, 2017).
34 Jon Delogu, *Fascism, Vulnerability, and Escape from Freedom* (Santa Barbara, California: Punctum Books, 2022).
35 Walter Laqueur (Ed.), *Fascism: A Reader's Guide: Analyses, Interpretations, Bibliography* (Berkeley and Los Angeles: University of California Press, 1976).
36 Martin Kitchen, *Fascism* (Houndmills, Basingstoke, Hampshire: Macmillan, 1976).
37 Avihu Zakai, *Jewish Exiles' Psychological Interpretations of Nazism* (Cham, Switzerland: Palgrave Macmillan, 2020).
38 Israel W. Charny, *Fascism and Democracy in the Human Mind: A Bridge between Mind and Society* (Lincoln, Nebraska: University of Nebraska Press, 2006).
39 Antonios Vadolas, *Perversions of Fascism* (London: Karnac Books, 2009).
40 Babak Fozooni, *Psychology, Humour and Class: A Critique of Contemporary Psychology* (Abingdon, Oxon: Routledge, 2020).
41 Frie, *Edge of Catastrophe.*
42 Neil McLaughlin, *Erich Fromm and Global Public Sociology* (Bristol: Bristol University Press, 2021).
43 Leighton Grist, *Fascism and Millennial American Cinema* (London: Palgrave Macmillan, 2018).
44 Richard Schacht, *Alienation* (London: Psychology Press, 2015 [1970]).
45 Christoph Henning, *Theories of Alienation: From Rousseau to the Present* (Abingdon, Oxon: Routledge, 2024).
46 Christopher J. Hewer and Evanthia Lyons (Eds), *Political Psychology: A Social Psychological Approach* (Hoboken, NJ: Wiley, 2018).
47 Terry D. Cooper, *Paul Tillich and Psychology: Historic and Contemporary Explorations in Theology, Psychotherapy, and Ethics* (Macon, GA: Mercer University Press, 2006).
48 Lars Tummers, *Policy Alienation and the Power of Professionals: Confronting New Policies* (Northampton: Edward Elgar, 2013).
49 James A. Tyner, *The Alienated Subject: On the Capacity to Hurt* (Minneapolis, MN: University of Minnesota Press, 2022).
50 R. Felix Geyer and David R. Schweitzer (Eds), *Theories of Alienation: Critical Perspectives in Philosophy and the Social Sciences* (Cham, Switzerland: Springer, 2012 [1976]).
51 See, e.g., Stephen Brookfield, "Overcoming Alienation as the Practice of Adult Education: The Contribution of Erich Fromm to a Critical Theory of Adult Learning and Education," *Adult Education Quarterly* 52, no. 2 (2002): 96–111; Deguchi, "Post-Truth Politics as a Pathology of Normalcy"; Enzo Lio, "Alienation as a Central Concept in Marxist and Frommian Humanism," Presentation at a German-Italian Seminar about *Die Marx Rezeption Erich Fromms*, Bologna, Italy, 17–19 February 1989, http://www.fromm-gesellschaft.eu/images/pdf–Dateien/Lio

_E_1989b.pdf; Sakurai, "The Socio-Psychological Base of Contemporary Fascism in the World of Liberal Democracy"; Mark K. Smith, "Erich Fromm: Alienation, Being and Education," in *The Encyclopedia of Informal Education*, 2002, http://www.infed.org/thinkers/fromm.htm; John F. Wozniak, "Alienation and Crime: Lessons from Erich Fromm," in Kevin Anderson and Richard Quinney (Eds), *Erich Fromm and Critical Criminology: Beyond the Punitive Society* (Urbana and Chicago: University of Illinois Press, 2000), 43–58.

52 Kevin Anderson and Richard Quinney (Eds), *Erich Fromm and Critical Criminology: Beyond the Punitive Society* (Urbana and Chicago: University of Illinois Press, 2000).

53 Lawrence Jacob Friedman, *The Lives of Erich Fromm: Love's Prophet* (New York: Columbia University Press, 2013).

54 Sakurai, *Political Theories of Narcissism.*

55 See the references cited in note 50: Deguchi, "Post-Truth Politics as a Pathology of Normalcy"; Lio, "Alienation as a Central Concept in Marxist and Frommian Humanism"; Sakurai, "The Socio-Psychological Base of Contemporary Fascism in the World of Liberal Democracy."

# 4 The Relevance of Fromm's Political Theory for Today

In chapters 1 and 2, an examination of the foundational principles of Fromm's theoretical framework has been conducted. The objective of this chapter is to provide a comprehensive elaboration of Fromm's theory, with the aim of making it applicable to contemporary twenty-first-century society. This endeavor seeks to facilitate an analysis of prevailing political issues and to propose solutions to them—however, it is important to note that Fromm's theoretical propositions are all derived from the twentieth century. Central to this elaboration are Fromm's theories of authoritarianism and narcissism. The subsequent analysis will demonstrate the functional relationship between his conceptions of authoritarianism and narcissism and his other fundamental conceptions, particularly as it concerns alienation within the ambit of free-market capitalism.

## A Frommian Theory of Narcissism

In what manner may we anticipate the manifestation of narcissism within social contexts characterized by alienation, as conceptualized by Fromm? Leveraging Fromm's social theory as a conceptual framework, this exploration elucidates the fundamental, functional linkage between alienation and narcissism within a social context. As previously discussed, in his social theory, narcissism functions as a character structure, both for society in general and for market-capitalist society specifically. This finding suggests that Fromm's conception of narcissism is indicative of mass society throughout the twentieth century and extending into the twenty-first century. Moreover, it suggests that the socioeconomic character structure of mass society is founded on market capitalism, a factor that has been identified as a contributing element to feelings of alienation. Additionally, Fromm's social theory of narcissism posits that contemporary society, coupled with the social functions of alienation, is engendering the "dialectic of narcissism," a developmental trajectory of social narcissism.[1]

The Frommian dialectic of narcissism postulates that, within the paradigm of market capitalism, human life is profoundly influenced by the narcissistic inclinations of individuals. However, these individuals are also compelled to transcend their own narcissistic tendencies. From a Frommian perspective,

DOI: 10.4324/9781003600398-5

this dialectic manifests in at least three ways: first, in the dichotomy between the necessity of narcissistic desires and the necessity of overcoming them; second, in the dichotomy between consumption and alienation; and third, in the dichotomy between democratic and fascist paths in terms of self-love and narcissism. With regard to the second issue, the dichotomy is construed as dialectical, on the grounds that the more people become dependent on consumption, the more alienation, the very condition that afflicts them, can become entrenched. This is due to the fact that the social function of consumption today largely stems from the idea of capital that underlies the market economy under capitalism. However, this dialectical process remains unconscious to individuals. A narcissistic sociocharacter structure fosters the development of narcissistic needs under the socioeconomic conditions of alienation, as the gratification of these needs is primarily derived from consumerism. Accordingly, in Fromm's social theory, both narcissism and alienation are intimately related, or more accurately, mutually reinforcing. From an ideological perspective, these two societal factors serve to reinforce the prevailing social order and bolster each other. On this basis, social narcissism follows a dialectical path.

### *Economic Narcissism*

As Fromm argues, the possession of "property" is emblematic of the fundamental human aspiration within the capitalist system, which perpetuates and reinforces a state of alienation.[2] In this social setting, narcissism is a significant hindrance to democracy due to the prevailing consumerist social conditions. Individuals seek to satisfy their narcissistic tendencies and foster a sense of contentment, known as the having mode, which necessitates narcissism through continuous adaptation to a market-driven society. In contemporary society, the satisfaction of one's personal needs, often referred to as "narcissism," is considered a key component of a marketing-oriented societal role. This approach has been demonstrated to address the dual objectives of fulfilling individual needs while contributing to societal benefits. Fromm therefore conceptualizes narcissism as an obstacle to the formation of a humanistic society that aspires to expand democratic principles. Fromm argues that the prevailing character structure fosters a "separateness and antagonism of individuals toward each other" and a "worship of industrial production."[3] These elements are at odds with democratic politics. In Fromm's view, human beings are confronted with the challenge of containing and subsequently overcoming narcissism.

In Fromm's social theory, the sociopathological functions of narcissism can be discerned in the economic dimension, especially in the combination of narcissism and alienation. This phenomenon is indicative of a narcissistic character structure that prioritizes self-promotion and the pursuit of personal gain, frequently at the expense of others, within the context of free-market systems—this tendency is conceptualized as *economic narcissism*.[4] Fromm argues that the free market is contingent on two factors: narcissism, defined as the desire to rationalize free-market mechanisms, and alienation, a social pathology engendered by capitalist free-market systems. In such circumstances, narcissism functions sociopathologically, fostering alienation.

The economic implications of narcissism can be illustrated as shown in Table 4.1. The concept of "humanity" in a negative sense, specifically narcissism, possesses its own distinct character structure. Narcissism, in its essence, can be conceptualized as an exploitation of others in the performance of its functions. In contrast to the narcissistic tendency, the concept of humanism entails self-love, which can be defined as a "productive orientation" that engenders effective and constructive interactions with others. Fromm's concept of "productive work" underscores the value of humanism in promoting meaningful contributions to society.[5] The concept of "productive activity" is defined as the capacity to engage with others through the medium of interpersonal relationships, underpinned by the ability to relate to others through love, and to "reach to [*sic*] the essence of things and processes" through reason.[6] However, it is important to note that societal progress is impeded by the pervasive influence of a narcissistic character structure. Liberal democracy is characterized by a narcissistic orientation, thereby fostering and being fostered by alienation, which is defined as the exploitation of others—human beings are regarded as objects of capital, designated as labor power, due to their reliance on machines and products.

In addressing the emergence of a political system that underlies the character structure of economic narcissism, Fromm elucidates the characterological transformation from the "hoarding orientation" to the "receptive orientation" during the twentieth century.[7] The crux of the discussion is that, while the former orientation was intertwined with the "exploitive orientation" in the nineteenth century, the latter orientation became increasingly intertwined with the "marketing orientation" in the twentieth century. Fromm's

*Table 4.1* The Frommian character structure of economic narcissism

| Negative forms of humanity and system | Orientations | Semantic meanings of the orientations |
|---|---|---|
| Humanity in the sense of narcissism | Narcissistic orientation | Exploitation of others |
| Humanity in the sense of self-love | Self-love orientation | Productive work (working together with others) |
| Liberal democracy | marketing orientation | Alienation (human beings as labor power and their dependence on machines and products) |

*Source:* modified Table 6.1, Sakurai, *Political Theories of Narcissism*, 191

work offers a compelling perspective on the evolution of capitalism, highlighting its transitions from a primarily exploitative economic model to one characterized by greater sophistication. This shift, as elucidated by Fromm, is accompanied by a transition in people's lifestyles, moving from a focus on material accumulation and consumption to a more refined and nuanced approach: "receiv[ing]... drink[ing] in ... [and] hav[ing] something new all the time" on a marketing level.[8] This suggests that the development of narcissism between the nineteenth and twentieth centuries was so substantial that society is now firmly rooted in a character structure characterized by narcissism. This phenomenon has enabled individuals to prioritize the acquisition of new possessions, a pursuit facilitated by the prevailing market society and its marketing for which they have needed the market society and its marketing-oriented strategies.

### *Political Narcissism*

If the mechanism of these economic functions of narcissism continues to thrive, as seen in Fromm's theory of narcissism, then it will be politically detrimental to Frommian democracy. In this case, politics is undergoing a pathological evolution based on malignant narcissism. In this context, the populace naturally demands politics that reduce the economic, asymmetrical balance of power that exists between the upper and middle classes and the working class under market capitalism, which forces individuals to satisfy their own lives solely through consumption. Paradoxically, their actions are propelled by a relentless pursuit of consumption, a phenomenon that is compounded by the forces of the market economy, which engender a pervasive sense of urgency. This urgency forces consumers to satiate their desires within the context of market capitalism. Consequently, the segment of the population that is discontented with the status quo is likely to demand political transformation. In a market society, individuals are theoretically endowed with the freedom to be autonomous. In practice, however, these individuals are not free to be independent because they are essentially incapable of living without dependence on the socioeconomic systems in place. Fromm illustrates this psychological state of society metaphorically as follows:

> Primary bonds once severed cannot be mended; once paradise is lost, man cannot return to it. There is only one possible, productive solution for the relationship of individualised man with the world: his active solidarity with all men and his spontaneous activity, love and work, which unite him again with the world, not by primary ties but as a free and independent individual. However, if the economic, social and political conditions on which the whole process of human individuation depends, [sic] do not offer a basis for the realisation of individuality in the sense just mentioned, while at the same time people have lost those ties which gave them security, this lag makes freedom an unbearable

> burden. It then becomes identical with doubt, with a kind of life which lacks meaning and direction. Powerful tendencies arise to escape from this kind of freedom into submission or some kind of relationship to man and the world which promises relief from uncertainty, even if it deprives the individual of his freedom.[9]

The fundamental assertion is that, within Fromm's sociotheoretical framework, socioeconomic conditions characterized by alienation—which are contingent on market-capitalist mechanisms—give rise to a pernicious form of group narcissism. This dynamic, in turn, engenders a downward spiral within society, perpetuating the cycle and giving rise to a political agenda that stands in direct opposition to the tenets of Frommian humanism. Fromm's social theory of narcissism elucidates that, in a political context, this collective narcissistic malignancy manifests through pathological political movements, such as racist chauvinism and extreme fanaticism, through a process he terms "social transference."[10] Within the theoretical scheme, however, the association between narcissism and fascism remains largely unexamined. This observation underscores the necessity for a systematic elucidation of the connection between these two theoretical components, which constitutes the crux of Fromm's theory of narcissism, for it to contribute meaningfully to the broader discourse on fascism.

In Fromm's social theory, the political functions of narcissism can be observed as well. In this theoretical framework, individuals exhibit a pathological dependence on one another for the gratification of their own sadomasochistic desires. This tendency is referred to as *political narcissism*, a term used to describe a pervasive sense of self-absorption within the political landscape.[11] In a political structure marked by an overreliance on narcissistic tendencies, a societal framework predicated on a political form of narcissism, individuals strategically exploit the strengths of others in a pathological relationship, driven by the pursuit of self-interest. This dynamic ultimately fosters the gratification of their own needs and the instigation of pathological politics. In such a context, individuals are permitted to prioritize their own self-interest, frequently at the expense of others, and to engage in manipulative behaviors to gain the acceptance and approval of their peers. This phenomenon, termed social narcissism, impedes the effective operation of democratic institutions. Within this paradigm, society engenders a pernicious form of narcissism, in which individuals perceive themselves as superior to others. This pathological desire is rooted in the fulfillment of their narcissistic needs. At times, it can also be associated with an authoritarian politics that masochistically relies on a charismatic political leader who promises people life satisfaction under the conditions of lost "primary bonds."[12] In summary, it is evident that this society is poised to evolve into an authoritarian social structure, a process that is facilitated by the presence of malignant narcissism, sadomasochistic symbiosis, and necrophilia. These phenomena serve to reinforce the authoritarian tendencies that are characteristic of such a societal structure.[13]

The conceptual framework for understanding political narcissism is delineated in Table 4.2. This phenomenon manifests in the political sphere, in most cases inciting chauvinist political movements that subsequently evolve into fascist politics. However, the phenomenon of political narcissism does not inevitably lead to the exacerbation of chauvinism or the rise of fascism. Instead, it always manifests in more subtle ways, assuming forms that are not readily apparent. Nevertheless, contemporary political movements have come to demonstrate a notable reliance on this narcissistic orientation. This form of narcissism frequently remains veiled by market-based democratic practices, a phenomenon that is especially evident in liberal democracies. In essence, this form of democratic politics inherently incorporates a narcissistic component, thereby signifying that contemporary fascism is, in a functional sense, supported by narcissism, which in turn sustains liberal democracy. It is imperative to recognize that the prevailing political orientation, which is predicated on the social conditions of a free-market economy, will continue to be shaped by the prevailing narcissistic orientation of our own character structure. It is only through a transformation of our character structure, from a narcissistic orientation to a self-love orientation, that we can truly hope to move beyond the confines of the social conditions of a free-market economy and toward a more equitable and sustainable political landscape. The marketing orientation that underlies liberal democracy is, by its very nature, formed on the basis of a narcissistic character structure.

The advent of fascist movements within liberal-democratic societies is frequently ascribed to particular social conditions that give rise to these ideologies. In accordance with a Frommian theory of political narcissism, authoritarian movements emerge in conjunction with a marketing orientation. The distinguishing factor between the authoritarian and marketing character structures is the extent to which the former is dependent on individuals, while the latter is contingent on entities, chiefly machines and products. In essence, these two phenomena are indistinguishable in terms of their functional characteristics, namely their pathological dependency and pursuit of objectives through the exploitation of surroundings. This is analogous to the semantic aspect of narcissism, which is typified by an inflated sense of self-importance and a preoccupation with one's own needs and desires. For

*Table 4.2* The Frommian character structure of political narcissism

| Negative forms of politics | Orientations | Semantic meanings of the orientations |
|---|---|---|
| Chauvinism | Narcissistic orientation | Exploitation of others |
| Fascism | Authoritarian orientation | Sadomasochistic symbiosis (dependence on others)<br>Necrophilia (destructiveness) |

*Source:* modified Table 6.1, Sakurai, *Political Theories of Narcissism*, 191

these reasons, the concept of *liberal-democratic* fascism is structurally intertwined with the character structure of narcissism.

When the character structures of both economic and political narcissism are examined from a dual perspective, then the emergence of phenomena can be anticipated as illustrated in Table 4.3. Within the framework of the narcissistic character structure, a parallel can be drawn between liberal democracy and fascism, as both demonstrate a comparable degree of construction. It is evident that both the authoritarian and marketing characters are founded on the narcissistic orientation characteristic of liberal democracies. The marketing orientation therefore exhibits certain fundamental aspects of authoritarianism. When viewed through this particular lens, liberal democracy can be interpreted as an internalization of the fascist, authoritarian orientation. However, liberal democracy is distinct from fascist types of political systems. In these societies, the authoritarian and marketing orientations are predicated on the character structure of narcissism, an orientation that is evident at both the individual and social levels. This orientation is typified by the leveraging of others to achieve personal objectives. If this is the case, then the sadomasochistic orientation is inherently implicated in the exploitation of others in liberal democracies, where individuals are compelled to prioritize their own market value as a means of subsistence. For this reason, sadomasochism emerges as a manifestation of the social conditions of alienation within the context of liberal democracy, despite the absence of an authoritarian origin.

In this section, I will examine the methodological significance of a Frommian theory that I have previously elaborated in the context of actual political scenarios. In consideration of the concept of fascism, it is essential to investigate the viability of employing the Frommian social theory of narcissism to analyze contemporary populist movements.. In order to facilitate comprehension, three relevant perspectives are hereby proposed for consideration: first, the application of a *from within*, internal viewpoint to illustrate

*Table 4.3* The two-dimensional Frommian character structure of economic and political narcissism

| Negative forms of humanity and political system | Orientations | Semantic meanings of the orientations |
|---|---|---|
| Humanity in the sense of narcissism | Narcissistic orientation | Exploitation of others |
| Liberal democracy | Marketing orientation | Alienation<br>(human beings as labor power and their dependence on machines and products) |
| Fascism | Authoritarian orientation | Sadomasochistic symbiosis<br>(dependence on others)<br>Necrophilia (destructiveness) |

*Source:* modified Table 6.1, Sakurai, *Political Theories of Narcissism*, 191

the mechanisms through which democratic systems deteriorate; second, two kinds of fascism, *political* and *economic*; third, the *pathological functions of a narcissistic character structure in a political dimension*. The initial perspective expounds upon the dialectical collapse of democracy. The second delineates economic fascism as fascist movements in the economic sphere that eradicate the democratic aspects of free markets and authoritatively legitimize their own economic activities through economic narcissism. Furthermore, it delineates political fascism as a political movement that deliberately dismantles the democratic tenets of society and employs a form of political narcissism to authoritatively legitimize its own political agenda.[14] The third sheds light on a mechanism that elucidates the pathological underpinnings of contemporary society and politics.

It is evident that the political system most pertinent to these three perspectives is indisputably liberal democracy, indicating that the United States is most analogous to a representative liberal democracy—not in the neoliberal sense, but rather in the sense of a sociopolitical system that perpetuates the social functions of alienation and narcissism. From these three perspectives, it is possible to reflect on US Trumpism and clarify its fascist orientations and functions using the Frommian social theory of narcissism as a conceptual lens. Indeed, it provides a valuable source of insight into the contemporary manifestation of fascism in the United States, a society characterized by a pervasive narcissistic culture. From this perspective, it is important to note that fascist social conditions bring about a dialectical transformation from an economic form of fascism (economic fascism) to a political form of fascism (political fascism). Economic narcissism, defined as a narcissistic desire to be liked by others in the free-market economy, is often unable to sufficiently meet its own needs because of the social structure of the market mechanism, which demands survival solely through the sale of oneself. This phenomenon can be attributed, in large part, to the law of economic fascism, a sociopathological mechanism that disrupts democracy from within through the exploitative free-market economy. Numerous individuals therefore encounter challenges in this highly competitive environment. It is evident that these individuals are not adequately meeting their narcissistic needs, and as a result, they are not leading fulfilling lives. In this case, the economic narcissism characteristic of the working class is transformed into a malignant form, giving rise to antagonistic feelings toward the ruling class. Concurrently, this narcissism induces racial xenophobia and heightened nationalistic sentiments. This phenomenon is precisely why economic narcissism is linked to political narcissism: a narcissistic desire to gratify one's sadomasochistic needs through incestuous dependence on others. For this reason, the phenomenon of working-class political narcissism is invariably dysfunctional, characterized by the transference of group narcissism to its narcissistic object, particularly to a political figure who pledges to ameliorate the prevailing social conditions of the working class and fulfill its aspirations.

This dynamic fosters the emergence of a fanatical, racist chauvinism through a process of social transference, whereby the narcissistic antagonism characteristic of working-class discontent is transferred to the political sphere. This fanatical movement subsequently transposes its inherent group narcissism onto a tangible narcissistic object, especially an authoritarian political figure who is tasked with regulating masochistic objects while concurrently fulfilling the narcissistic aspirations of masochistic individuals. This process is how political fascism is instigated. The majority of individuals within this demographic remain unaware of the fact that their actions ultimately serve to bolster the interests of the economic elite, despite the fact that their elected officials are often drawn from the same economic sector. This phenomenon can be further elucidated by observing that both the leaders of economic and political fascism are typically affiliated with the ruling class—within the context of the United States, it can be argued that the general public is, albeit unconsciously, providing tacit endorsement to an economic form of fascism, albeit indirectly through their support for a political manifestation of this ideology embodied by Donald Trump, a quintessential representative of the economic elite. This phenomenon helps elucidate why and how American society has twice been poised for dramatic political change. These nationwide transformations were the result of a social form of transference that had spawned racist, chauvinistic group psychologies. These psychologies were transferred to Trump, who successfully exploited and manipulated people and their racist xenophobia based on narcissistic antagonism to gain national control over them, thereby satisfying his narcissism. This can be understood as a manifestation of the two recent dramatic political shifts of US society from an economic level of fascism to a political level of fascism.

## A Frommian Theory of Authoritarianism

What sociotheoretical inferences can be drawn from a Frommian theory of economic narcissism? What are the implications of this theory for social and political theory? A salient sociopathological feature identified by the theory pertains to the notion that fascism is indicative of the prevailing social conditions within contemporary market societies. In a system where the emergence of fascist politics is anticipated under the conditions of free-market capitalism, narcissism operates in tandem with alienation, concurrently inducing authoritarian tendencies involving sadomasochistic symbiosis and necrophilia. In liberal democracies, however, this kind of pathological politics does not simply mark the political form of a state or a government as a result of political mobilization. In the systems of liberal democracy, this concept refers to the lessons of everyday life that are disciplined by time and property. Specifically, it refers to "contemporary disciplined, workaday daily life."[15] In such social conditions, fascist movements flourish, particularly in the context of *labor market authoritarianism*, where individuals as labor power are subjected to manipulation by authoritarian, sadomasochistic political power in conjunction with alienation functions. Additionally, *workplace authoritarianism* engenders a sense of confinement to disciplined, quotidian working life. In this way, there is an increasing reliance on machines and products, while concomitantly nurturing narcissism as an unconscious human desire for support of the free market and its essential mechanisms.

### *Labor Market Authoritarianism*

Labor market authoritarianism is identifiable in a "Frommian social theory of narcissism," manifesting primarily in the forms of economic and political narcissism.[16] This can be attributed to the market's self-serving inclination to prioritize its own economic interests, resulting in a self-fulfilling cycle of authoritarianism. The populace of this need has been observed to exhibit tendencies consistent with narcissism, characterized by unconscious pursuit of self-aggrandizement at the expense of others. This behavior is perpetuated in a manner that contributes to the perpetuation of the market, and the individuals in question appear to be dependent on this dynamic for their sense of self-esteem and fulfillment. This phenomenon is due to the liberal-democratic systems that are prevalent in their society. These systems necessitate a reliance on machines for survival and are oriented toward marketing. Consequently, individuals find themselves in a state of dependency, effectively transitioning into the labor force. In this social state, the labor market exhibits its own arbitrary needs, built on the unconscious sadomasochistic desire to gain control over others and to feel powerful by transferring one's own weakness to authority. According to its own sadomasochistic inclinations, it manifests authoritarian character traits. As such, the labor market is inherently authoritarian, and its raison d'être is revealed exclusively through authoritarianism. The market's fundamental nature is revealed through its authoritarian mechanism. In summary, the labor market can be regarded as an illustration of socioeconomic mechanisms that operate through the two-dimensional character structure of economic and political narcissism. The market absorbs and exploits people's discipline for its own benefit, while the labor operates through the exploitation of others to sell oneself at the highest possible price. Concurrently, both parties engage in a sadomasochistic dynamic of mutual dependence, thereby fortifying their bond.

In the context of contemporary markets, it is widely accepted that, in liberal societies, especially those adhering to neoliberal economic principles, the market is effectively subject to the influence of substantial global and international corporations—transnational corporations (TNCs) or multinational corporations—including prominent world fund and investment banking groups.[17] This suggests that a significant proportion of the global workforce is affiliated with these corporations, either directly or indirectly, and is, as a result, inextricably linked with their corporate governance, whether consciously or unconsciously. This phenomenon, characterized by a self-destructive propulsion of these corporations and their management practices, merits further examination and analysis. This observation underscores a pivotal realization: the market's operation does not strictly adhere to the laws of supply and demand. Instead, it is more accurately influenced by the needs and preferences of TNCs.[18] It is hypothesized that under these arbitrary market conditions, liberal democracy becomes oligarchic rather than democratic. This transformation, therefore, entails a shift from democracy—a political rule of the power of the people (democrats)—into oligarchy—a rule of the power of certain groups (TNCs) (oligarchs).[19] However, it is crucial to acknowledge the formidable challenges in resisting this form of oligarchic politics, particularly given the pervasive influence of corporate governance within the domain of TNCs. This phenomenon is further compounded by the asymmetrical positioning of workers within the international political landscape, thereby exacerbating the difficulty of resisting the influence of these corporate entities.[20] These facts demonstrate the potential for the observation of certain authoritarian, pathological functions within contemporary market mechanisms. Thus, the labor market is regarded as operating under oligarchic principles.

The authoritarian nature of the labor market is evident from the above analysis. It is therefore hypothesized that the workplace functions in a similar manner. In contemporary society, individuals frequently find themselves compelled to adhere to consistent daily routine, a circumstance that is particularly pronounced within the context of the labor market. The free market, predicated on capital, requires a robust degree of discipline on the part of individuals, thereby ensuring their compliance with the temporal demands of the market. Fromm says:

> In industrial society time rules supreme. The current mode of production demands that every action be exactly "timed," that not only the endless assembly line convey or belt but, in a less crude sense, most of our activities be ruled by time. In addition, time not only is time, "time is money." The machine must be used maximally; therefore the machine forces its own rhythm upon the worker.[21]

In this social context, individuals endeavor to impose self-discipline in accordance with the imperatives of "time." In accordance with the prevailing mechanisms of time, all elements within the workplace undergo a transformation according to the requirement of the "mode of production." As previously stated, the labor market operates in accordance with its authoritarian demands, which stem from the sadomasochistic aspirations of TNCs and the labor force. From this perspective, the dynamics of the workplace are profoundly influenced by labor market authoritarianism, particularly in a manner that satiates its economic-narcissistic inclinations. In this context, the daily work of people is largely standardized in terms of discipline, regardless of the genres of "jobs."[22] In a liberal democracy, the lives of individuals are subject to stringent temporal and material constraints, thereby giving rise to a "contemporary disciplined, workaday daily life." Individuals often find themselves constrained to prioritize their professional lives exclusively over their personal ones. This is due to the fact that the workplace serves as the foundation for their existence and the labor market determines their overall worth in accordance with authoritarian mandates. As a result, individuals are unable to break free from the shackles of a life that is predetermined by the workplace. The populace is compelled to engage in self-destructive behaviors and to satisfy their own narcissistic proclivities by adhering to the tenets of workplace authoritarianism. However, they often remain unaware of the social obligations that the workplace imposes upon them, a failure that can have deleterious consequences.

As such, the political manifestation of liberal democracy is more apt to comprise an authoritarian character structure, wherein individuals engage in sadomasochistic interdependence within the mechanisms of narcissistic exploitation and the labor market. The political system thus functions more rationally within the mechanisms of the capitalist free market. In a liberal democracy, authoritarianism thrives not only in the political sphere but also in the economic and quotidian realms, particularly in the labor market and the workplace. However, at the subsequent level, the presence of authoritarian social elements becomes challenging to discern. This can be attributed to the prevalence of democratic social conditions, which are widely deemed the antithesis of authoritarian and fascist political systems. In the social context of liberal democracy, the main problem is the absence of discernible authoritarian orientations in practice. For this reason, it is imperative to ascertain the underlying factors that influence these orientations within the context of a liberal democracy.

Fromm's conception of narcissism is characterized by its inherent internalization of the philosophical and sociotheoretical concept of alienation, thereby fulfilling its functions in a sociotheoretical dimension rather than in a mere psychoanalytic framework. From this perspective, two types of narcissism can be delineated on a sociotheoretical level: economic narcissism, based on the marketing orientation; and political narcissism, based on the authoritarian orientation. These two social pathologies are inextricably interwoven in such a way that authoritarian needs are rather provoked by a marketing character structure. From this perspective, it is possible to perceive authoritarianism even in the sphere of the free-market economy. In this regard, liberal democracy has been observed to be more or less associated with authoritarian/fascist movements. That is to say, authoritarian character structures have been demonstrated to serve as a solid basis for fascism.[23]

The fundamental sociotheoretical significance of fascism in liberal democracy is precisely workplace authoritarianism, which rests on labor market authoritarianism. This authoritarian character structure compels individuals to engage in sadomasochistic self-discipline as labor power, conforming to the demands of the free market—a system from which escape is arduous. One of the most efficacious ways to address these pathologies of liberal democracy is to resist authoritarian repression in seemingly democratic practice. In this context, democracy appears as a "rebellious act," signifying a persistent endeavor to liberate oneself from the authoritarian constraints that legitimize the pathological mechanisms of workplace and labor market authoritarianism under the guise of democracy.[24]

### *Corporatism and Bureaucracy*

A Frommian theory that has been elaborated upon in this book should be consistent with an examination of the neoliberal type of society, especially the United States. However, the theory has not yet been adapted to social democracies on the same side of the liberal spectrum. What are the specific characteristics of this type of society, categorized as social-democratic or socialist-democratic societies? It is my position that corporatism is one of the most prominent social systems. It is a commonly held belief that Nazism signaled the demise of the tradition of German corporatism that had been in place until the Weimar era.[25] Due to the following reasons, however, this does not impede the interpretation of modern German history in a linear fashion. First, it is conceivable that the theoretical combination of Fromm's characterological conceptions can characterize both Nazism and German societal corporatism, irrespective of whether they never coexisted or are irreconcilable. Second, it is entirely feasible to recognize societal and state versions of corporatism along the same characterological line. Moreover, it is both irrelevant and, arguably, impossible to disassociate the entirety of the Nazi period from any other facets of modern German history from an ingenious historical standpoint that perceives Nazism as a discrete event in the past. For instance, in certain theories of fascism, Nazism is regarded as a manifestation of fascism (and Fascism) in the sense of the dialectical problem that a certain form of liberalism or socialism paradoxically evolves into fascist nationalism. The phenomenon is exemplified by specific political structures at the governmental level that are categorized as fascism, such as Italian Fascism and even US Trumpism. The pejorative appellation "National Socialism" aptly encapsulates the essence of this dialectic.[26] In this context, the following critical response to Antonio Costa Pinto, to whom reference was made above, is pertinent:

> A sense that we are missing something in neglecting corporatism is clearly an aspect of his restiveness. Although Italy was central to corporatist discussion, Germany was not, so better encompassing the interchange over corporatism can help us place the range of experiment on the new Right in better proportion. By implication, it has been teleological thinking, including privileging Nazi Germany excessively, that has kept us from doing so. Corporatism has been neglected both because Nazism, racism, expansionism, and war have come to seem quintessential and because, despite a great deal of interest and hype at the time, it never amounted to much practice.[27]

As David Roberts contends, corporatism can undoubtedly function as a pivotal element in the far-right political landscape, regardless of temporal or geographical constraints—however, a thorough historical investigation into this phenomenon is not pursued in this particular book. This inquiry can be approached from a theoretical angle with minimal historical content, as the book focuses on a sociopsychological analysis of the character structure of our society. In a nutshell, it is postulated that Nazism and German corporatism coexisted in a state of inextricable intertwining, with the latter ultimately becoming the prevailing social structure within contemporary Germany—from this perspective, the two phenomena can be regarded as inseparable components within the broader context of German history. Contemplating Nazism invariably entails contemplating German corporatism, and vice versa. It is conceivable that the structure of German corporatism has functioned as a defining characteristic of modern Germany, particularly since the twentieth century.

Within the framework of Nazism–German corporatism, these two social and political organizations are theorized to be interconnected by the amalgamation of Fromm's characterological conceptions. This theoretical combination elucidates the alignment of societal and state versions of corporatism. While this book does not address Nazism or corporatism, it asserts that Fromm's conception of authoritarianism offers insights into their *sociopsychological underpinnings* from a pathological angle—focusing not on their social structures themselves. Thus, certain modifications of Fromm's conception of authoritarianism are directed toward a sociopsychological, ideological analysis of contemporary postfascist, authoritarian movements that have proliferated in select social-democratic, corporatist societies.

From these perspectives, it is not an exaggeration to say that some core aspects of social and political mechanisms, regardless of place, are even enlivened by authoritarianism—the focus of this discussion is on the operation of an authoritarian orientation in bureaucratic systems. It is hypothesized that Germany has operated on this basis, maintaining this approach over the past 150 years. It can be argued that, on the positive side of modernity, the German authoritarian-bureaucratic orientation was ironically a factor in the rapid achievement of the democratization of postwar Germany.[28]

At this juncture, it is necessary to reformulate Fromm's theory of authoritarianism, incorporating his conceptions of narcissism and bureaucracy. In this reformulation, I will demonstrate, from a Frommian perspective, that postfascist movements in Germany spring from a group-narcissistic antagonism toward strangers, characterized by their authoritarian character structures. This social character is predicated on an ingrained fear of erratic life that has been in existence and has been operated by the German bureaucratic orientation, reinforced by the Weberian "authoritarian mentality" that can be enriched by the Frommian authoritarian personality.[29] This pervasive sense of entrenched fear falls into at least two distinct classifications: historical and psychological. The former phenomenon is explainable by the concept of "German angst" in the historical sense.[30] The German authoritarian-bureaucratic character under scrutiny herein builds on the war trauma of the Germans, thereby spawning a series of fears that rise and fall in chronological order: these include their "postwar angst" and "moral angst," the "Cold War angst" of nuclear war, "modern angst existing during the 1950s and 1960s" about the uncertainty of modernization, and "democratic angst."[31] These apprehensions collectively represent "a future-oriented emotion," stemming from a sense of uncertainty. The latter phenomenon is explained by the concept of "uncertainty avoidance," as described by social psychologist Geert Hofstede.[32] This particular form of fear-based psychological behavior operates through the avoidance of uncertainty per se. The primary rationale for its operation is its psychological mechanism of not causing fear and anxiety, a mechanism by which the German people can evade uncertainty.[33]

In this book, "bureaucracy" is used to refer to an orientation that internalizes "necrophilia." This use of the term "bureaucracy" is distinct from its conventional use and serves to distinguish the concept from the broader context of bureaucracy.[34] In essence, this approach can be characterized as an abstract, automatic, and mechanical psychological perspective on human life. Germany, in its entirety, is *predominantly* characterized by this approach to life and, to a lesser extent, by the marketing orientation that a neoliberal society embodies. This orientation is evident in both *qualitative* and *quantitative* aspects. However, it is important to note that the former society is also intertwined with the marketing character. In other words, the German system places a greater emphasis on bureaucracy in both *quality* and *quantity* compared to market systems, while the neoliberal system places a significant reliance on the latter. A comparison of the German and neoliberal *character structures* reveals both quantitative and qualitative differences.

### *The Authoritarian Personality*

Fromm's conceptualization of authoritarianism is primarily evident in his three books: his early work, *Studien über Autorität und Familie* (Studies on Authority and Family) (1936);[35] his seminal work, *Escape from Freedom* (1941); and his later work, *The Heart of Man* (1964).[36] His examination of the concept is structured into three distinct levels:

- The initial focus of this study is the sociopsychological underpinnings of authoritarianism, with an emphasis on the social functions of the Western patriarchal family system;
- "Sadomasochism," in which individuals exhibit a pathological dependence on each other, demonstrates a reluctance to face loneliness and engage in authoritarian desires due to an inability to endure psychological solitudes, and their personalities are shaped by symbiotic relationships;[37]
- The following three orientations are associated with the concept under discussion: "necrophilia," "narcissism," and "incestuous tie."[38]

Fromm expounds on the evolution of authoritarianism as follows. The father, who was granted patriarchal authority on a national level, was combined with "sadomasochism," which created the sociopsychological basis for fascism, that is, Nazism. The sadomasochistic character is structured to form a symbiosis. Thus, within social contexts that perpetuate the fragmentation of the self, individuals are compelled by the aspiration to establish connections through what Fromm terms a "secondary bond." This phenomenon arises as a result of the profound psychological distress experienced in an atomized state of being.[39] The subjects in question have been observed to transition out of this psychological state of mind, specifically by relating themselves to the secondary bond. Although Fromm subsequently applied the concepts of "necrophilia," "narcissism," and "incestuous tie,"[40] these psychological concepts have yet to be effectively incorporated into his conception of authoritarianism. Instead, it appears that the concept of necrophilia has become more closely linked to bureaucracy, while the concepts of narcissism and incestuous ties have become more associated with authoritarianism.

### *The Bureaucratic Orientation*

The most symbolic connotation of Fromm's conception of bureaucracy is provided by his other conception of necrophilia. However, when it comes to the concept of necrophilia, it is evident that Fromm's analysis lacks a clear distinction between the authoritarian and bureaucratic orientations. Nevertheless, he appears to have achieved a substantial degree of success in conceptualizing bureaucracy by employing the concept to provide nuanced insights into the intricacies of character development. This phenomenon is most transparently observed in *The Heart of Man*. According to Fromm, the necrophilous orientation is characterized by a lack of emotional warmth, a sense of detachment, and a commitment to upholding established "law and order."[41] The subsequent section will delve deeper into these character traits, exploring the subject's attraction to darkness and night, and orderliness, as well as their propensity for obsession and pedantry. Fromm maintains that individuals who exhibit a combination of these traits do not genuinely love life. Instead, they are driven by a desire to "correct division," perceiving this as justice. Their mechanistic approach to life consequently results in an "intellectual–abstract" mode of thinking.[42] It can be argued that these characteristics serve to control everything in terms of the intense fear and anxiety that leads to, and is embedded and structured within, the necrophilous orientation that requires the bureaucratic orientation.

It is conceivable that, in his work on bureaucracy, combined with the concept of necrophilia, Fromm transitioned his focus from the sociopsychological issues of socialist, corporatist societies to those of the infrastructure of the free market. In doing so, he embarked on an investigation into the qualitative similarities between corporatism and the free-market economy. In this regard, it would be worthwhile to catch a glimpse of how both of their bureaucratic character structures are intertwined with the market mechanism, particularly in neoliberal societies. Despite this theoretical shift, however, I posit that the fundamental purpose of utilizing the necrophilous orientation as a heuristic is to elucidate certain salient sociopsychological features of socialist corporatism that demand an extensive degree of bureaucracy, insofar as it aims to delineate the character structure of bureaucracy.

Overall, the necrophilous character is typified by an *abstract* and *automatic-mechanical* approach to human life, thereby revealing the psychological underpinnings of the bureaucratic orientation. This configuration is widely regarded as the archetypal manifestation of bureaucracy's systemic and organizational framework. In this context, the manner in which individuals interact with one another becomes a secondary concern. The primary focus is on the effectiveness of the system and organization as a whole, irrespective of the impact these abstract, automatic, mechanical processes might have on interpersonal relationships and human dignity. From Fromm's perspective, bureaucracy stands in direct opposition to humanism, as exemplified by his term "bureaucratic industrialism" as a counterpoint to "humanist industrialism."

### *The Frommian Authoritarian-Bureaucratic Orientation*

The integration of these two conceptions and narcissism remains a subject of ongoing inquiry. The focal point of this attempt is the manner in which the mechanisms of social narcissism intertwine with sadomasochistic symbiosis and an abstract, automatic-mechanical approach to human life under market capitalism. In the majority of advanced countries today, authoritarianism operates predominantly within the framework of a capitalist market economy, leading to an inevitable narcissistic orientation at the socioeconomic level. This indicates that contemporary society is characterized by the operation of authoritarian mechanisms within narcissistic social functions, thereby driving the market mechanism. Concurrently, the bureaucratic orientation that fortifies bureaucracy is firmly entrenched in this milieu, frequently concomitant with authoritarianism manifesting as an authoritarian-bureaucratic character. The authoritarian orientation thus serves to strengthen bureaucracy in itself. In a Frommian theory, these three sociocharacterological functions are interdependent, operating in a dynamic interplay within the context of contemporary market society. This interplay is characterized by the influence of two overarching social functions: narcissism and bureaucracy. It is acknowledged that there is a lack of sufficient interconnection between the concepts of narcissism and bureaucracy, given their tendency to function in largely distinct ways. This assertion is indeed valid; however, it is imperative to acknowledge the predominance of bureaucratic structures in contemporary market societies. As a result, narcissism is conducive to the bureaucratic orientation, and vice versa. This phenomenon is particularly evident in societies such as Germany, a society that is characterized by an authoritarian-bureaucratic character structure.

It appears that a combination of the aforementioned orientations will shed light on the sociopsychological underpinnings of both the Nazi police state and German corporatism, as previously referenced. It is arguable that in a society emerging from an amalgamation of these two social systems, in a Frommian approach, the sadomasochistic human relationships that the society immanently internalizes will instigate an authoritarian politics by transferring the group's narcissistic needs to a charismatic political leader who slakes the society's desires *to maintain its bureaucratic order*. A character structure specific to this type of society can be identified here as *a Frommian authoritarian-bureaucratic orientation*. Within this character structure, the profound fear of unknown elements within the social sphere leads to the rigidification of the bureaucratic system, thereby influencing all aspects of society, including human personal relationships. As a result, foreigners and political minorities, who are often perceived as unknown and unspecified entities, are naturally ostracized and occasionally detested within the social context. For this reason, the enactment and administration of a new law by the bureaucracy for the use of "unspecified" beings and things in German society is imperative. Moreover, the prevailing conditions of mass society, characterized by profound social isolation, necessitate the development of a secondary bond with authority by means of bureaucratic orientations that are both sadistic and destructive and obedient and functional. It is hypothesized that this phenomenon underlies the emergence of fascist politics in contemporary societies that are firmly rooted in a Frommian authoritarian-bureaucratic orientation.

## Postfascism and Fromm's Political Theory

In what ways does the Frommian theory developed herein demonstrate its relevance in the analysis of political phenomena related to fascism, such as populism? It is noteworthy that Fromm himself rarely employed the term "populism." Instead, he demonstrated a predilection for the term "fascism," particularly in the context of its association with the character structure of mass society.[43] This association pertains to the various social contexts that are pertinent to the issues of populism. From this perspective, the scope of fascism is indisputably embedded within modern and contemporary society. However, it is important to acknowledge that the contemporary era differs considerably from the period to which Fromm's conception of mass society pertains. This observation underscores the limitations of employing Fromm's social theory to analyze twenty-first-century society. This book, therefore, emphasizes the potential of the concept of fascism to elucidate contemporary sociopathological phenomena within a *historical continuum*. The book proposes that the Frommian critical social theory of narcissism, as expounded in this chapter, will offer a novel perspective on contemporary sociopolitical conditions in liberal democracies, as illustrated by Enzo Traverso's sociopsychological conception of postfascism. To this end, the terms "fascism" and "postfascism" will be employed to illuminate the sociopsychological underpinnings of present-day US society. A salient implication of this exploration is that fascism in our society represents economic and political fascism emerging as postfascist movements.

### *Postfascism*

The term "postfascism" is believed to have emerged in the aftermath of World War II. Recently, Traverso has put flesh on the bones of the concept of the word through a genealogical analysis.[44] The foundational essence of the idea is articulated as follows: "postfascism belongs to a particular regime of historicity—the beginning of the twenty-first century—which explains its erratic, unstable, and often contradictory ideological context, in which antinomic political philosophies mix together."[45] In essence, postfascism can be characterized as a political movement that aims to destroy democracy "from within" by adopting the fundamental principles of fascism.[46] In other words, postfascism is driven by a pathological desire to dismantle the foundational processes of democratic deliberation, a pursuit facilitated by the metamorphosis of the theoretical underpinnings of traditional fascism. This metamorphosis preserves what has been termed a "plebiscitary model of democracy," thereby ensuring the continued subversion of democratic norms and values.[47]

The issues associated with postfascist politics, a corollary of liberal democracy, can be elucidated through an examination of Fromm's social theory, emphasizing the narcissistic character structures prevalent in society. This theory transcends traditional disciplinary boundaries, merging elements from multiple fields of study. By centering on sociopsychological determinants, it sheds light on the nature of far-right political movements as an extension of a fascist political paradigm. Frommian works, particularly those addressing contemporary far-right issues, offer a nuanced perspective by emphasizing the sociopsychological underpinnings of fascism.[48] Fromm's theoretical framework offers a provocative perspective, positing democracy and fascism as dialectical constructs.[49] Fromm's social theory, especially his theory of narcissism, meticulously examines postfascist forms of politics within the context of liberal democracies.

The considerable promise of the concept of "postfascism" in the far-right context remains underestimated in current scholarship.[50] According to Traverso, postfascism encapsulates the prevailing impolitical and postideological trends observed within contemporary right-wing populist and right-wing extremist movements. The ensuing discussion will delve into the salient aspects of Traverso's conception of postfascism. While Germany can be defined by postfascism, no one has yet rigorously explicated the country's politics in the current discourse on the concept. This dearth of analysis can be ascribed to two factors: the recent emergence of the term "postfascism" in academic discourse and the necessity for a more robust and sustained analytical understanding of the concept, which remains in its nascent stages. The prevailing discourse of populism has dominated the field of political theory and related areas, overshadowing the exploration of postfascism. The primary rationale for the applicability of the political concept is that the fundamental elements of the far right in Germany are embodied by the concept of populism, which can be substituted with that of postfascism—these concepts exhibit significant overlap in many respects. I contend that the conceptual framework of postfascism offers a more efficacious means of comprehending far-right politics within the context of liberal democracies. This approach underscores the qualitative (e.g., ideological) distinctions that set these societies apart.

A critical distinction must be made between postfascism and neofascism. In her foundational work, Anna Cento Bull expounds on this distinction, positing that "neo-fascism" signifies radical, political, and ideological movements that draw upon the "revolutionary nature of fascism" while upholding "radical and uncompromising views.".[51] Neofascism can thus be conceptualized as a postwar political movement that, in its revolutionary nature, uncompromisingly seeks the destruction of the core facets of modernity, including humanism, under bureaucratic systems as well as under conditions of postwar and contemporary mass society. A hallmark of neofascism is its commitment to radical political transformation, underpinned by the consent of the masses, in favor of a wartime fascist ideology. From this perspective, the survival of the neofascist movement appears to be contingent not on its political positioning but rather on its ability to adapt to and take advantage of the adverse aspects of modernity. This suggests that, from a pragmatic perspective—as opposed to a formalistic one—neofascism is not aligned with the positive aspects of modernity, particularly democracy, which is known to foster humanism, but rather with its negative aspects, such as bureaucracy, which works against humanism, particularly in the context of postwar and contemporary mass society. The distinguishing characteristics of postfascism and neofascism are as follows: the former's *involuntary* and *unpredictable* dynamics, which take on a *postideological* and *impolitical* complexion; and the latter's voluntary, ideological, and political nature. In this respect, each of these ideologies occupies a diametrically opposed position. Within the framework of a comparative analysis of these three forms of fascism, postfascism can be conceptualized as a quantitatively *mild form* of fascism that emerges within the context of mass society under advanced capitalism. In summary, as posited by a Frommian theory I have elaborated, a specific strain of postfascism has emerged within the German far-right movement, thriving under capitalist social structures characterized by authoritarian bureaucracy and social narcissism.

The following discourse endeavors to present a comprehensive overview of the concepts of "fascism" and "postfascism." From a historical standpoint, Germany offers some of the most intriguing insights into these movements. The genesis of these two movements is multifaceted, involving the social conditions of capitalism, mass society, and bureaucracy.[52] Germany's historical trajectory through fascism laid the foundation for a significant shift toward postfascism, which is characterized by the prominent influence of the German New Right. This movement elegantly encapsulates the Frommian authoritarian-bureaucratic orientation, rendering it a captivating subject to explore. From a Freudian perspective, the notion that humans possess an innate authoritarian tendency is intriguing, and the extent of this tendency ultimately determines its manifestation.[53]

At this juncture, I will demonstrate how the reformulation of Fromm's theory of authoritarianism can illuminate the existence of two distinct postfascist political movements in Germany. The initial type is characterized by the actions of far-right groups, including Pegida and Hooligans against Salafists (HoGeSa), and is designated as the agitation type of postfascism. The second type is driven by far-right parties, such as the Alternative für Deutschland (AfD), and individuals with far-right leanings and is designated as the propagandist type of postfascism.[54] These phenomena are frequently interpreted as manifestations of right-wing populism or right-wing extremism. I will argue that both phenomena exhibit narcissistic antagonism, especially toward refugees and immigrants, an aggressive impulse that has been induced by their chronic fear of specific immigrants and foreign residents—this assertion is based on a Frommian authoritarian-bureaucratic character that has been formulated above. The ensuing discourse will elucidate the notable parallels between right-wing populism and right-wing extremism within the context of German far-right politics. Additionally, the discussion will illuminate the substantial distinction between neofascism and some other forms of extremist right-wing movements. Furthermore, a novel categorization of these two types of far-right politics *in liberal democracies* is proposed as exemplary postfascist politics. However, a paucity of consensus exists among scholars regarding the categorization of populism, whether right-wing or left-wing, in the same lineage as fascism.[55] Conversely, the concept of extremism is, to a certain extent, conceptualized by prominent scholars as falling within the ambit of fascism.[56] Additionally, some theorists of fascism regard both right-wing populism and right-wing extremism in liberal democracies as postfascist, a corollary of liberal-democratic politics.[57] It is noteworthy that in the United States, the phenomenon of Trumpism—which is viewed as a manifestation of right-wing populism within a neoliberal society—is frequently interpreted as the "alt-right" (abbreviation for the "alternative right").[58] A thorough examination of this term reveals a striking resemblance to the concept of the German New Right.

### *The Sociopsychological Basis of Postfascism in Germany*

#### *Application of a Frommian Authoritarian-Bureaucratic Orientation*

A discussion of postfascism can be approached through the lens of two distinct socioeconomic systems: neoliberalism and corporatism. While the former is sometimes associated with postfascist politics in relation to economic class struggle,[59] the specific association with the latter remains unclear. In the context of contemporary populist movements in Germany, where a liberal democracy implements corporatism, the analysis of *immigration* and *refugee-related issues* is crucial to elucidate the factors that have led to the emergence of these movements in the nation.[60] The theoretical underpinnings of these issues are believed to be rooted in social systems of authoritarian bureaucracy, which are closely associated with social-democratic corporatism in Germany.

In the subsequent section, the sociopsychological underpinnings of the German neofascist and postfascist right wing will be examined, with a particular focus on five representative German right-wing groups and individuals who exhibit pronounced far-right tendencies. The results of this analysis will be presented in Table 4.4. As previously mentioned, two categories of postfascist political movements in Germany can be distinguished: the agitation type of postfascism, exemplified by Pegida and HoGeSa, and the propaganda type of postfascism, represented by the AfD and the party's current and future diehard supporters. However, this distinction is merely nominal, as both categories are fundamentally classified within the overarching category of German postfascism.

In the context of neo-Nazism, the object of veneration is unambiguously Nazi leaders. Key terms employed for political propaganda include the German noun *das Volk*, signifying the English concept of "folk" or "nation," and its adjective *völkisch*, denoting "national." These terms were strategically utilized by the Nazi regime.[61] The radical objective of these groups is to establish a right-wing utopia through the exclusion or expulsion of immigrants and refugees from the living space referred to as *das Volk*.[62] The social psychology of the neo-Nazis is predicated on anxiety regarding the unspecified and unknown, inducing an excruciating fear that manifests as "xenophobia."[63] These elements are perceived by them as impediments to their existence and the existence of their society, which is founded on an authoritarian-bureaucratic orientation reminiscent of Fromm's theories. It is evident that prominent German right-wing extremist parties, such as the National Democratic Party of Germany (NPD) and the Free German Workers' Party (FAP), are representative of neo-Nazis in Germany.[64]

Pegida, a right-wing extremist group based in Germany, places significant emphasis on the concept of *das Volk*. This term is employed in conjunction with the term *völkisch*, a term frequently utilized in propaganda and a matter of significant concern.[65] The ideological objective of the group's movement is to exclude or purge German immigrants and refugees, particularly those

*Table 4.4* The sociopsychological underpinnings of the neofascist and postfascist right-wing movements in Germany

| *Types of fascism* | *neofascism* | | *postfascism* | | |
|---|---|---|---|---|---|
| Right-wing groups | neo-Nazis | | New Right | | |
| | National Democratic Party of Germany (NPD) | Free German Workers' Party (FAP) | Pegida | AfD | PPL |
| Non-fascist categorization | right-wing extremism | √ | √ | right-wing populism | unclear |
| Objects of worship | Nazi leaders (concrete) | √ | *das Volk* (abstract) | √ | unclear |
| Representative words used for propaganda | *das Volk*, *völkisch* | √ | √ | *Sozialpatriotisch*, *völkisch* | unclear |
| Goals | foundation of a national utopia (radical) | √ | exclusion or purge of immigrants & refugees (conservative) | √ | √ |
| Social psychologies | fear of the unspecified (xenophobia) | √ | √ | √ | √ |

of Muslim heritage.[66] This is predicated on the agitation group's belief that these individuals pose a threat to the continued existence and cultural integrity of the German nation. However, a thorough examination uncovers that the sociopsychological underpinnings of Pegida are analogous to those of neo-Nazis, stemming from an intense fear of the undefined.

The political party AfD shares with the Pegida movement a focus on the concept of *das Volk*. However, a closer examination of the party's propaganda reveals a broader vocabulary that extends beyond the terms *völkisch* and *das Volk*.[67] The party utilizes a number of adjectives that denote political conservatism, including *sozialpatriotisch* (social patriotic).[68] However, it is also noteworthy that the AfD appears to have a policy of excluding or purging *die Ausländer* (foreigners) from Germany, a term that is used to refer to specific immigrants and refugees.[69] From this perspective, the movement is based on the sociopsychological fear of the unspecified.

The general populace that lends its support to political parties such as the AfD and their leaders, and which harbors far-right dispositions, can be influenced and manipulated by the party's political strategies and propaganda. This dynamic can manifest in the veneration of a shared object, the propagation of each other's ideologies in a manner analogous to that of their leaders, and the adoption of slogans that bear resemblance to those employed by far-right movements. Despite self-identifying as fundamentally different from neo-Nazis and the Nazis, these individuals can be influenced and manipulated in a manner similar to that of the groups mentioned above.[70] However, their actions are not solely influenced by the leadership, but rather by their personal experiences and behaviors, which are rooted in a social psychology characterized by acute anxiety about the unknown. This anxiety fosters a type of fear that leads to xenophobia, thereby justifying the creation of social scapegoats.

It is evident that the aforementioned far-right movements share notable similarities in their ideological composition. Nevertheless, a salient distinction emerges between neo-Nazis and other far-right groups with regard to the veneration of specific Nazi leaders.[71] As previously mentioned, neofascism signifies a radical, political, and ideological movement that maintains a strong adherence to the "revolutionary nature of fascism," while concurrently upholding "radical and uncompromising views." This ideological orientation is further characterized by its *voluntarism*, *ideological* purity, and *political* commitment. This ideological orientation is exemplified by neo-Nazis, who embody the aforementioned characteristics.[72]

Conversely, postfascism is distinctly delineated from neofascism in terms of its *involuntary* and *unpredictable* dynamics, as well as its *postideological* and *impolitical* character, as articulated by Traverso. Instead, it operates through the "upholding of a plebiscitary model of democracy," thereby *unconsciously* undermining democratic politics from within. This postfascist stance is exemplified by prominent far-right groups such as the AfD and the agitation-oriented organizations, including the Pegida and HoGeSa movements. Their actions, lacking in radicalism, appear spontaneous and are devoid of any coherent ideological underpinnings. A plausible hypothesis is that these groups are predicated on simple dissatisfaction with life, manifesting in far-right political orientations.

A salient point of this discussion is the observation that both neofascism and postfascism employ similar mechanisms to disseminate their ideological objectives and to influence *societal psychology*. This phenomenon is indeed elucidated in the Frommian theory of authoritarianism. The *sociopsychological* underpinnings of both German neofascism and postfascism are characterized by their authoritarian-bureaucratic orientation, whereby the deeply ingrained fear of unspecified societal elements in a social dimension strengthens the country's bureaucratic systems, thereby influencing all aspects of society, including human interpersonal relationships. This dynamic engenders a societal environment in which foreigners and political minorities are often perceived as unknown and unspecified, leading to their ostracism, and at times, loathing and abhorrence. It is evident that both movements exhibit a striking disregard for the sociopsychological factors, as outlined above, that shape political realities, thereby adopting characteristics reminiscent of far-right ideologies.

A thorough examination of the right-wing elements that have come to define neofascism and postfascism in Germany reveals a particular configuration that emerges, as illustrated in Figure 4.1.1. Neofascism, as embodied by the neo-Nazi movement, is characterized by meticulous preparation, signifying an acute awareness of the congruence between its actions and its inherent nature, particularly with regard to the voluntary dynamics of neofascist politics. Moreover, it assumes a distinct form due to its ideological and political components. In contrast, postfascism can be characterized as an *ad hoc*, uncontrollable movement due to its involuntary and unpredictable dynamics, stemming from a lack of self-knowledge regarding its own nature. However, this characteristic does not exert a determining influence on postfascist politics, which takes an ambiguous form shaped by its postideological and impolitical nature. Nevertheless, this fact is inconsequential for postfascist politics, which takes an ambiguous form shaped by its postideological and impolitical nature. The political movements known as the AfD and Pegida, along with their respective supporters, have been classified as falling under the umbrella of fascist ideology.

A salient aspect of this phenomenon pertains to the sociopsychological underpinnings of both German neofascism and postfascism, which are characterized by a *Frommian authoritarian-bureaucratic character structure*. This orientation serves as a determining factor in their fundamental modes of being and acting. In Germany, the employment of the term *besorgte Bürger* (concerned citizens) has proven to be a remarkably efficacious catalyst for eliciting politically salient reactions from individuals who embody

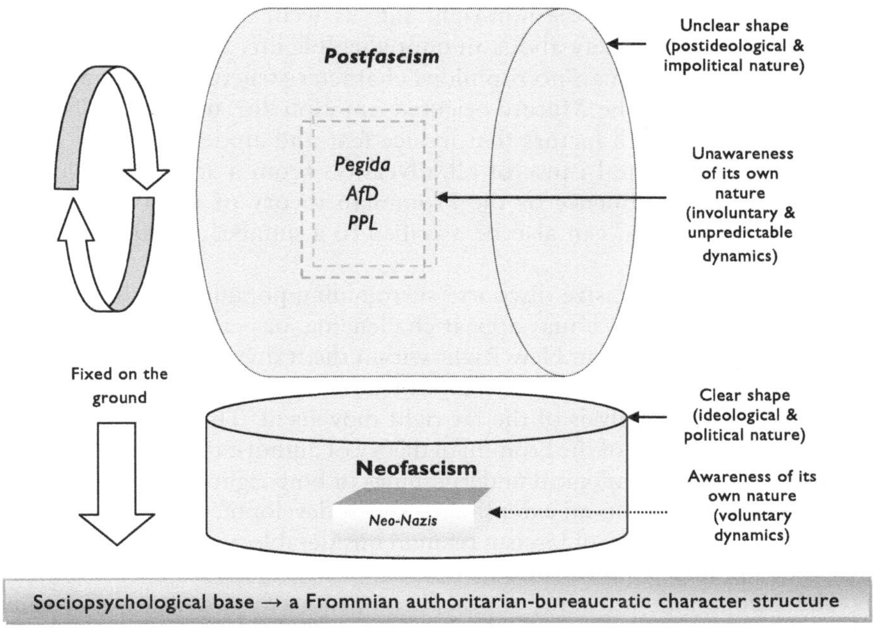


*Figure 4.1* The two Frommian sociopsychological structures of German far-right politics including its New Right movement

this character structure, particularly within the nation's right-wing milieu. These individuals adeptly navigate the political landscape by delineating the full spectrum of possibilities, thereby circumventing the elicitation of anxiety and fear.[73] In essence, this phenomenon aligns with a Frommian authoritarian-bureaucratic orientation, where a primal fear is evaded through two interwoven mechanisms. Firstly, there is an authoritarian tendency characterized by a sadistic desire to control others and a masochistic need for power. Secondly, there is a highly structured bureaucratic operation that utilizes an abstract and mechanical approach to human life, effectively eliminating erratic aspects without inducing worry.

Finally, it is imperative to pose a provocative question: does the character structure delineate solely the far right in Germany? For instance, it appears that the concept of "strangers" can be substituted with "far-right individuals," and the social psychological concept of "fear of the unknown" can be replaced with "fear of the far right."[74] Irrespective of the question of whether the slogan and the object of purge are separate entities, the German authoritarian-bureaucratic social character that engenders group-narcissistic hostility toward specific groups or figures functions in excluding or eliminating them on the non-right side as well, insofar as it similarly generates extreme anxiety about an unpredictable life, a morbid dread that springs from the German necrophilous character structure maintaining its own bureaucracy. The "future-oriented emotion for uncertainty" operates by eliminating all factors that induce fear and anxiety, thereby eradicating the fundamental cause of all adversity. From a sociopsychological perspective, the pertinence of the Frommian theory of authoritarianism, distinct from fascism, can also be ascribed to a number of leftist political orientations.[75]

In light of the pervasive discourse surrounding populism in the humanities and social sciences, it may appear challenging, or perhaps even unorthodox, to assess the German New Right within the framework of postfascism. However, it must be noted that the postfascism approach is not inherently unsuitable for the analysis of the far-right movement. This assertion is supported by the findings of the Frommian theory of authoritarianism, which elucidates the sociopsychological underpinnings of both right-wing populist and extremist phenomena as an extension of fascist developments. Consequently, the conceptual category of fascism retains considerable pertinence in examining contemporary populism and extremism.

The sociopathological and political phenomenon of posfascism in Germany is the result of the country's authoritarian and bureaucratic social character, which has led to a group-narcissistic hostility toward strangers, such as refugees, immigrants, and foreigners. This animosity is deeply rooted in the German populace's pervasive anxiety and apprehension regarding life, which have been engendered by their necrophilous orientation, thereby underpinning the bureaucratic system that is intrinsic to German society.

### *Problems with Fromm and Frommian theories*

Fromm's social theory does not account for the remarkable proliferation of financial markets and the consequent rise of global corporations to the extent that they have attained in the contemporary era. This perspective diverges from the contemporary interpretation of the concept of "free market" as it is currently understood. Instead, it refers to the dynamics that operated within mass society during the mid-twentieth century. Nevertheless, it is evident that his theory continues to offer a valuable lens for understanding the underlying causes of twenty-first-century social pathologies, particularly the prevalence of authoritarian orientations within democratic societies. The archetypal nature of these two examples, drawn from the contexts of the United States and Germany, has been thoroughly examined. However, it must be acknowledged that the socioculturally intricate nature of contemporary issues, intricately interwoven with transnational phenomena such as transnational corporations (TNCs) and social networking sites (SNS), might not be fully captured by a purely Frommian sociocharacterological perspective. As a result, the employment of alternative theoretical frameworks becomes imperative. The modification of Fromm's theory is essential to illuminate the relevance of its own theoretical framework. Adhering rigidly to the principles of Fromm's original theory may hinder the ability to fully explore its implications and potential contributions to the broader sociocultural landscape.

## Notes

1 Takamichi Sakurai, *Political Theories of Narcissism: Towards Self-Reflections on Knowledge and Politics from the Psychoanalytic Perspectives of Erich Fromm and Fujita Shōzō* (Zurich: LIT Verlag, 2018), Ch. 6, Sect. 6.3.2.5; Sakurai, "The Socio-Psychological Base of Contemporary Fascism in the World of Liberal Democracy," at 150.
2 Fromm, *To Have or To Be?*, 63.
3 Fromm, *Greatness and Limitations of Freud's Thought*, 53–54.
4 Sakurai, "The Socio-Psychological Base of Contemporary Fascism in the World of Liberal Democracy," 150; Sakurai, "A Frommian Perspective on the Socio-Psychological Structure of Post-Fascism in Liberal Democracies", at 185, 189.
5 See, e.g., Fromm, *Escape from Freedom*, 23; 1971[1947], 45.
6 Fromm, *Man for Himself*, 102; *To Have or To Be?* 74.
7 Fromm, *The Sane Society*, ch. 5.
8 Fromm, *The Sane Society*, 136.
9 Fromm, *Escape from Freedom*, 36–37.
10 Fromm, *The Heart of Man*; cf. Sakurai, *Political Theories of Narcissism*, "The Socio-Psychological Base of Contemporary Fascism in the World of Liberal Democracy," "A Frommian Perspective on the Socio-Psychological Structure of Post-Fascism in Liberal Democracies."
11 Sakurai, "The Socio-Psychological Base of Contemporary Fascism in the World of Liberal Democracy," 150; Sakurai, "A Frommian Perspective on the Socio-Psychological Structure of Post-Fascism in Liberal Democracies," 185, 189.
12 Fromm, *Escape from Freedom*, 36; see Sakurai, "The Socio-Theoretical Relevance of Erich Fromm's Psychoanalytic Conception of Narcissism," at 18–19.
13 Fromm, *The Heart of Man*; Erich Fromm, *The Anatomy of Human Destructiveness* (New York, Chicago and San Francisco: Holt, Rinehart and Winston, 1973). It is imperative to underscore that authoritarianism does not merely signify an "orientation"; rather, it is a consequence of prevailing political needs. (see Sakurai, "The Socio-Theoretical Relevance of Erich Fromm's Psychoanalytic Conception of Narcissism," 13).
14 See Sakurai, "The Socio-Psychological Base of Contemporary Fascism in the World of Liberal Democracy," 153.
15 Sakurai, *Political Theories of Narcissism*, 192.
16 Sakurai, "A Frommian Perspective on the Socio-Psychological Structure of Post-Fascism in Liberal Democracies," "The Socio-Theoretical Relevance of Erich Fromm's Psychoanalytic Conception of Narcissism."
17 William K. Carroll, *The Making of a Transnational Capitalist Class: Corporate Power in the 21st Century* (London: Zed Books, 2010); Terry Hathaway, "Neoliberalism as Corporate Power," *Competition & Change*, 24, nos. 3–4 (2020): 315–37; Dieter Plehwe, Bernhard J. A. Walpen, and Gisela Neunhöffer, *Neoliberal Hegemony: A Global Critique* (Abingdon, Oxon: Routledge, 2006); William I. Robinson, *Global Capitalism and the Crisis of Humanity* (New York: Cambridge University Press, 2014); William I. Robinson and Jeb Sprague, "The Transnational Capitalist Class," in Mark Juergensmeyer, Saskia Sassen, Manfred B. Steger, and

Victor Faessel (Eds), *The Oxford Handbook of Global Studies* (New York: Oxford University Press, 2018), 309–27. The "transnational capitalist class" (TCC) is of particular interest here (Carroll, *The Making of a Transnational Capitalist Class*; William I. Robinson, *A Theory of Global Capitalism: Production, Class, and State in a Transnational World* (Baltimore, MD: Johns Hopkins University Press, 2004); Robinson and Sprague, "The Transnational Capitalist Class;" Leslie Sklair, *The Transnational Capitalist Class* (Oxford: Blackwell, 2011).

18 Robinson, *A Theory of Global Capitalism*, *Global Capitalism and the Crisis of Humanity*; Robinson and Sprague, "The Transnational Capitalist Class."

19 Shelly Gottfried, *Contemporary Oligarchies in Developed Democracies* (Cham, Switzerland: Palgrave Macmillan, 2019); Adrian Pabst, *The Demons of Liberal Democracy* (Cambridge: Polity, 2019); Žarko Paić, *Neoliberalism, Oligarchy and Politics of the Event: At the Edge of Chaos* (Newcastle upon Tyne: Cambridge Scholars Publishing, 2020).

20 Carroll, *The Making of a Transnational Capitalist Class*; Robinson, *A Theory of Global Capitalism*, *Global Capitalism and the Crisis of Humanity*.

21 Fromm, *To Have or To Be?* 104.

22 It is noteworthy that the term "job" is defined as "piece of work," thus underscoring the contemporary concept of "division of labor," particularly evident in manufacturing processes where workers engage in disparate tasks while maintaining a uniform pace. This phenomenon potentially provides a valuable lens through which to interpret Fromm's thematic focus on time.

23 Fromm, *Escape from Freedom*, *The Heart of Man*; see Sakurai, "A Frommian Perspective on the Socio-Psychological Structure of Post-Fascism in Liberal Democracies."

24 Markus Pausch, *Demokratie als Revolte: Zwischen Alltagsdiktatur und Globalisierung* (Baden-Baden: Nomos, 2017); Markus Pausch, "Democracy Needs Rebellion: A Democratic Theory Inspired by Albert Camus," *Theoria: A Journal of Social and Political Theory* 66, no. 161 (2019): 91–107.

25 See, e.g., Klaus Neumann, "Inter-War Germany and the Corporatist Wave, 1918–1939," in Antonio Costa Pinto (Ed.), *Corporatism and Fascism: The Corporatist Wave in Europe* (Abingdon, Oxon: Routledge, 2017), 124–43; Howard J. Wiarda, *Corporatism and Comparative Politics: The Other Great "Ism"* (Abingdon, Oxon: Routledge, 2015 [1997]).

26 For an examination of interpretations of Trumpism in accordance with this dialectic, see, e.g., Sakurai, "A Frommian Perspective on the Socio-Psychological Structure of Post-Fascism in Liberal Democracies"; Traverso, *The New Faces of Fascism*.

27 David D. Roberts, *Fascist Interactions: Proposals for a New Approach to Fascism and Its Era, 1919–1945* (New York and Oxford: Berghahn, 2016).

28 The substantiation of these claims would be greatly facilitated by the presence of empirical evidence.

29 David Beetham, *Max Weber and the Theory of Modern Politics* (Cambridge: Polity Press, 1985), 124, 168; cf. Max Weber, *Gesammelte Politische Schriften* (Tübingen: J.C.B. Mohr, 1988).

30 See, e.g., Frank Biess, *German Angst: Fear and Democracy in the Federal Republic of Germany* (New York: Oxford University Press, 2020); Michael Pickering and Thomas Kehoe (Eds), *Fear in the German-Speaking World, 1600–2000* (New York: Bloomsbury).

31 Biess, *German Angst*, 818.

32 Geert Hofstede, *Culture's Consequences: International Differences in Work-Related Values* (Newbury Park, CA: Sage, 1980).

33 This phenomenon can be conceptualized as the psychological mechanism of "escape from freedom," as articulated by Fromm: Fromm, *Escape from Freedom*.
34 For an expanded discussion on the bureaucratic orientation and necrophilia, refer to the section entitled "The bureaucratic orientation."
35 Fromm, "Sozialpsychologischer Teil," 77–135; Erich Fromm et al., "Zweite Abteilung: Erhebungen," in *Studien über Autorität und Familie*, 229–469.
36 A plethora of recent publications have emerged on the subject of conception. Among these recent publications, the following works merit particular attention: Braune, *Erich Fromm's Revolutionary Hope*; Thorpe, *Necroculture*; Charles Thorpe, "Escape from Reflexivity: Fromm and Giddens on Individualism, Anxiety, and Authoritarianism," in Joan Braune and Kieran Durkin (Eds), *Erich Fromm's Critical Theory: Hope, Humanism, and the Future* (London: Bloomsbury Academic, 2020).
37 Fromm, *Escape from Freedom*, Chs 5–6.
38 Fromm, *The Heart of Man*, Chs 3–5.
39 Fromm, *The Heart of Man*, 141.
40 Fromm, *The Heart of Man*, Chs 3–5.
41 Fromm, *The Heart of Man*, 40–41.
42 Fromm, *The Heart of Man*, 57.
43 See, e.g., Fromm, *Escape from Freedom*, *To Have or To Be?*; cf. Sakurai *Political Theories of Narcissism*, ch. 6, Sects. 6.4.2, 6.4.3.
44 Traverso, *The New Faces of Fascism*.
45 Traverso, *The New Faces of Fascism*, 7.
46 Traverso *The New Faces of Fascism*, 5.
47 Traverso *The New Faces of Fascism*, 28.
48 Douglas Kellner, "Donald Trump, Media Spectacle, and Authoritarian Populism," *Fast Capitalism* 14, no. 1 (2017): 75–87; Kellner, "Donald Trump as Authoritarian Populist," 71–82; Michael A. Peters, "'The Fascism in Our Heads': Reich, Fromm, Foucault, Deleuze and Guattari—the Social Pathology of Fascism in the 21st Century," *Educational Philosophy and Theory* 54, no. 9 (2020): 1276–84; Sakurai, "The Socio-Psychological Base of Contemporary Fascism in the World of Liberal Democracy," "A Frommian Perspective on the Socio-Psychological Structure of Post-Fascism in Liberal Democracies," "The Socio-Theoretical Relevance of Erich Fromm's Psychoanalytic Conception of Narcissism."
49 Fromm, *Escape from Freedom*, *To Have or To Be?*; cf. Sakurai, *Political Theories of Narcissism*, "The Socio-Psychological Base of Contemporary Fascism in the World of Liberal Democracy," "A Frommian Perspective on the Socio-Psychological Structure of Post-Fascism in Liberal Democracies."
50 For the concept of postfascism, see Traverso, *The New Faces of Fascism*, ch. 1; cf. Sakurai, "A Frommian Perspective on the Socio-Psychological Structure of Post-Fascism in Liberal Democracies." The employment of the term "post-fascism," most frequently written as "post-fascism," has been traced back to the immediate post-World War II era. However, it is only since the 1990s that this term has been employed with the rigidity and consistency that is characteristic of contemporary scholarship. The term has been utilized by numerous scholars in the humanities, most notably by the eminent theorist of fascism Roger Griffin. He employed the term in a specific context, namely to describe the Italian far-right political party Alleanza Nazionale: Roger Griffin, "The 'Post-Fascism' of the Alleanza Nazionale: A Case Study in Ideological Morphology," *Journal of Political Ideologies* 1, no. 2 (1996): 123–45; cf. Carlo Ruzza and Stefano Fella, *Re-Inventing the Italian Right: Territorial Politics, Populism and 'Post-Fascism'* (Abingdon, Oxon: Routledge, 2009). The term was later conceptualized by the Romanian philosopher Gáspár

Miklós Tamás, for example, who defined it as follows: Gáspár Miklós Tamás, "On Post-Fascism: The Degradation of Universal Citizenship," *Boston Review: A Political and Literary Forum*, 1 June 2000, http://bostonreview.net/world/g-m-tamas-post-fascism; Gáspár Miklós Tamás, "What Is Post-Fascism?," *openDemocracy*, 31 September 2001, https://www.opendemocracy.net/en/article_306jsp. Recently, Enzo Traverso, whom I have previously cited, advanced a more rigorous theoretical framework in his book: Traverso, *The New Faces of Fascism*, ch. 1.

51 Anna Cento Bull, "Neo-Fascism," in R. J. B. Bosworth (Ed.), *The Oxford Handbook of Fascism* (Oxford: Oxford University Press, 2009), 586–605, at 586. This perspective aligns with that of the preeminent theorist of fascism, Roger Griffin.

52 For a more thorough examination of this topic, see Sakurai, "A Frommian Perspective on the Socio-Psychological Structure of Post-Fascism in Liberal Democracies"; Traverso, *The New Faces of Fascism*; cf. Fromm, *Escape from Freedom*, *To Have or To Be?*

53 Sigmund Freud, "Introductory Lectures on Psycho-Analysis (Part III)," in James Strachey (Ed. and Trans.), *The Standard Edition of the Complete Psychological Works of Sigmund Freud*, vol. 16 (1916–17) (London: Hogarth Press, 2001).

54 In addressing the subject of agitation type, the focus will be on Pegida.

55 See, e.g., Sheri Berman, "Populism Is Not Fascism: But It Could Be a Harbinger," *Foreign Affair*, 95, no. 6 (2016): 39–44; Finchelstein, *From Fascism to Populism in History*; Cas Mudde and Cristóbal Rovira Kaltwasser, *Populism: A Very Short Introduction* (New York: Oxford University Press, 2017).

56 See, e.g., Stephen E. Atkins, "Introduction," in Stephen E. Atkins (Ed.), *Encyclopedia of Modern Worldwide Extremists and Extremist Groups* (Connecticut: Greenwood Press, 2004); Klaus von Beyme, "Right-Wing Extremism in Post-war Europe," in Klaus von Beyme (Ed.) *Right-Wing Extremism in Western Europe* (Abingdon, Oxon: Routledge, 2013), 1–18; Andrea Mammone, Emmanuel Godin, and Brian Jenkins, "Introduction," in Andrea Mammone, Emmanuel Godin, and Brian Jenkins (Eds), *Varieties of Right-Wing Extremism in Europe* (Abingdon, Oxon: Routledge, 2013), 1–15.

57 Sakurai, "A Frommian Perspective on the Socio-Psychological Structure of Post-Fascism in Liberal Democracies"; Traverso, *The New Faces of Fascism*.

58 See, e.g., George Hawley, *The Alt-Right* (New York: Oxford University Press, 2019); Patrik Hermansson, David Lawrence, Joe Mulhall, and Simon Murdoch, *The International Alt-Right: Fascism for the 21st Century?* (Abingdon, Oxon: Routledge, 2020); Shannon.E. Reid and Matthew Valasik, *Alt-Right Gangs: A Hazy Shade of White* (Oakland, California: University of California Press, 2020).

59 Sakurai, "A Frommian Perspective on the Socio-Psychological Structure of Post-Fascism in Liberal Democracies"; cf. Traverso, *The New Faces of Fascism*.

60 See, e.g., Takamichi Sakurai, "Minshushugi ni okeru media to rondan: Doitsu no nyūsu magajin ni miru kami-baitai no gendaiteki jōken" (The Functions of Media and Opinion Leaders in Contemporary Democracy: The Present State of Paper-Based Opinion Magazines, as Evidenced by German News Magazines), *Jōkyō* (fifth ed.), 1, no. 1 (2018): 8–22; Hans Vorländer, Maik Herold, and Steven Schäller, *PEGIDA and New Right-Wing Populism in Germany* (Cham, Switzerland: Palgrave Macmillan, 2018).

61 See, e.g., Günther B. Ginzel, *Hitlers (Ur)enkel: Neo-Nazis, Ihre Ideologien und Aktionen* (Düsseldorf: Droste, 1981).

62 See, e.g., Rand C. Lewis, *The Neo-Nazis and German Unification* (Westport, Connecticut and London: Praeger, 1996).

63 Gerard Braunthal, *Right-Wing Extremism in Contemporary Germany* (Houndmills, Basingstoke, Hampshire: Palgrave Macmillan, 2009); Lewis, *The Neo-Nazis and German Unification*.

64 See, e.g., Michael Minkenburg, "The New Radical Right in the Political Process: Interaction Effects in France and Germany," in Martin Schain, Patrick Hossay, and Aristide R. Zolberg (Ed.), *Shadows Over Europe: The Development and Impact of the Extreme Right in Western Europe* (New York: Palgrave Macmillan, 2002), 245–68.

65 Pegida, "28. Jahrestag des Mauerfalls," *Pegida*, 9 November 2017, https://www.pegida.de/news/28-jahrestag-des-mauerfalls.html; Vorländer et al., *PEGIDA and New Right-Wing Populism in Germany*.

66 Pegida, "28. Jahrestag des Mauerfalls"; Vorländer et al., *PEGIDA and New Right-Wing Populism in Germany*; cf. DGB Jugend, *AfD und Pegida: Die neue Rechte* (Blickpunkt: nur "besorgte Bürger?" June 2016), http://www.jugend.dgb.de.

67 Cathérine Colliot-Thélène, "Populism as a conceptual problem," in Gregor Fitzi, Juergen Mackert, and Bryan S. Turner (Eds), *Populism and the Crisis of Democracy: Volume 1: Concepts and Theory* (Abingdon, Oxon: Routledge, 2019), 17–26; Ayhan Kaya, *Populism and Heritage in Europe: Lost in Diversity and Unity* (Abingdon, Oxon: Routledge, 2020); Joseph Sterphone, "'Mut zu Deutschland!': On the Populist Nationalism of the Alternative für Deutschland," in Fernando López-Alves and Diane E. Johnson (Eds), *Populist Nationalism in Europe and the Americas* (New York: Routledge, 2019), 99–115.

68 Frauke Petry, "Wir sind der Stachel im Fleisch," Philip Eppelsheim (Intvw.), *Frankfurter Allgemeine Woche*, 20 (2018): 27–29; cf. Christoph Butterwegge, Gudrun Hentges, and Gerd Wiegel, *Rechtspopulisten im Parlament: Polemik, Agitation und Propaganda der AfD* (Frankfurt am Main: Westend Verlag, 2018).

69 Alice Weidel, *Widerworte: Gedanken über Deutschland* (Kulmbach: Plassen Verlag, 2019); cf. Sterphone, "Mut zu Deutschland!"

70 See, e.g., Jan Herman Brinks, *Children of a New Fatherland: Germany's Post-War Right-Wing Politics* (London: I.B. Tauris, 2000); Jan Herman Brinks, "Germany's New Right," in Jan Herman Brinks, Stella Rock, and Edward Timms (Eds), *Nationalist Myths and Modern Media: Contested Identities in the Age of Globalization* (London: I.B. Tauris, 2006), 125–38. In this context, the paradoxical view of Brink's book that "'right-wing' norms and institutions were preserved under a 'left-wing' banner" is of particular interest (Brinks, *Children of a New Fatherland*, 51). With regard to the vernacular in Germany, consult, e.g., Siegfried Jäger, "Political Discourse: The Language of Right and Left in Germany," in Patrick Stevenson (Ed.), *The German Language and the Real World: Sociolinguistic, Cultural, and Pragmatic Perspectives on Contemporary German*, revised ed. (Oxford: Clarendon Press, 1997), 233–57. He asserts: "[p]ublic discourse in contemporary Germany is predominantly colored by conservative and right-wing ideologies and ideas, especially as regards everyday thinking and debate" (Jäger, "Political Discourse," 233).

71 Braunthal, *Right-Wing Extremism in Contemporary Germany*; Lewis, *The Neo-Nazis and German Unification*.

72 Braunthal, *Right-Wing Extremism in Contemporary Germany*; Lewis, *The Neo-Nazis and German Unification*.

73 DGB Jugend, *AfD und Pegida*; Christian Fuchs, *Nationalism on the Internet: Critical Theory and Ideology in the Age of Social Media and Fake News* (Abingdon, Oxon: Routledge, 2019), ch. 6.

74 For instance, consider the profound aversion exhibited by the far left toward the far right, as elucidated by Dan Hough and Dan Keith in their seminal work, "The

German Left Party: A Case of Pragmatic Populism," in Giorgos Katsambekis and Alexandros Kioupkiolis (Eds), *The Populist Radical Left in Europe* (Abingdon, Oxon: Routledge, 2019). In contrast, Óscar García Agustín, *Left-Wing Populism: The Politics of the People* (Bingley: Emerald Group Publishing, 2020).

75 Fromm posits the hypothesis of the existence of left-wing authoritarianism: Erich Fromm, *The Working Class in Weimar Germany: A Psychological and Sociological Study* (Cambridge, MA: Harvard University Press, 1984).

# Conclusion

## Is Fromm Still Relevant?

From a reflective perspective, we have examined Fromm's main contributions and considered their relevance for our twenty-first-century society. Fromm's birth occurred in the final year of the nineteenth century, and he lived until the late twentieth century. His thought was therefore reflective of the historical period of those centuries. It is evident that Fromm's perspective, characterized by his era, could not encompass the conceptualization of our AI society today. His thinking and writing predate 1980, the year of his passing, and it has been nearly half a century since his death. Moreover, Fromm's contributions have historically received minimal attention from academic circles. This is primarily due to the prevailing sentiment among scholars of a disapproving nature toward his theoretical work. It is reasonable to hypothesize that a considerable number of individuals within the academic community continue to exhibit skepticism regarding the contemporary relevance of Fromm's contributions to scholarship.

What inferences can be drawn from this perspective that reveals disadvantageous facts about Fromm? As previously discussed, Fromm's thought is widely regarded as being highly pertinent to the analysis of populist and authoritarian politics in present-day society. Moreover, it proposes a theoretical framework relevant to postfascism, a Traversian concept of authoritarian politics in the contemporary era. However, these strengths are essentially confined to scholarly contributions. It must be recognized that the fundamental purpose of Fromm's oeuvre is not restricted to the aforementioned subjects. Instead, it endeavors to enhance the spiritual quality of people's lives, a pursuit that is of paramount importance. In this context, the true relevance of Fromm's work lies beyond the confines of the academic realm, particularly within the domains of the humanities and social sciences. Yet, the prevailing conceptualizations of these disciplines nowadays often fail to adequately prioritize direct contributions to people and society. The fundamental objective of these institutions is to facilitate scholarship, a pursuit that is largely dissociated from the realities of our daily lives. In these academic fields, indirect societal contributions are predominantly perceived as incidental outcomes. Humanities scholars nowadays, for the most part, demonstrate a notable lack of concern for such ancillary benefits.

DOI: 10.4324/9781003600398-6

In light of this consideration, the rationale behind the apparent disdain for Fromm within academic circles can be attributed to the classification of his thought as mundane knowledge. Additionally, the simplicity of his writing is regarded as rendering it ill-suited for academic scrutiny.[1] Nonetheless, his dialectical theory remains opaque, as has been previously observed. It is noteworthy that the majority of extant scholars do not find it appealing due to its seemingly ordinary nature; their interests are typically focused on specific subjects. These facts have been overlooked even by scholars specializing in Fromm, possibly because they also perceive Fromm through the lens of their academic expertise. In my estimation, the optimal approach to reading Fromm is as a novice reader, with the objective of comprehending his thought, while setting aside methods and questions that are relevant to academia.[2] This approach is believed to facilitate a more nuanced comprehension of Fromm's thought.

From this perspective, the question arises as to whether Fromm's relevance lies in offering ordinary knowledge that facilitates a more profound understanding, for example, of love for others. While there is some veracity to this claim, it is crucial to acknowledge that this does not represent the primary function of his theory. Its objective is to analyze society, identify societal problems, and propose solutions to address them. In this sense, Fromm's theory is interpretive and descriptive. However, it is important to note that these practical roles transcend the purview of interpretive theory. The discernible presence of normative functions within his theoretical contributions is a salient feature.[3] Nevertheless, the prevailing pertinence of Fromm's thought lies chiefly in its capacity for critical social theory, which is regarded as having two primary functions: namely, diagnosis and prescription.[4] His critical social theory employs medical epistemology and functions by examining society, identifying social pathologies, and prescribing remedies.[5]

This prompts the question of the present-day status of critical theory. It is evident that the primary focus of this approach is on normative constructions rather than on diagnostic and prescriptive objectives. Jürgen Habermas has developed a theory of communicative action to establish normative foundations, thereby contributing to the conceptual framework of deliberative democracy. Axel Honneth's contributions to the field of normative theory are marked by the introduction of a theory of recognition, drawing upon psychoanalysis as a theoretical framework. Claus Offe proposes a basic income as a solution to the adverse effects of capitalism, thereby facilitating the realization of the normative standards required by contemporary democracy. Rainer Forst employs Kantian practical philosophy to elucidate the capabilities of rational beings and attain several fundamental normative objectives of justification. In her oeuvre, Rahel Jaeggi underscores several foundational modern traditions in German philosophy and proffers a proposal for an alternative to capitalist social conditions.

Critical theory has become exclusively associated with normative theory. Honneth uses psychoanalysis for prescriptive purposes; yet, it does not appear that his objective is to prescribe solutions.[6] Forst's approach appears to prioritize the conceptual underpinnings of justification over the practical value of the theory itself.[7] Conversely, Fromm's relevance rather lies in the utilization of his theory for diagnostic and prescriptive purposes. This book indeed seeks to explore the contemporary relevance of Fromm in terms of critical theory in diagnostic and prescriptive contexts.

Fromm's primary relevance lies not in his contributions to normative foundations but rather in his potential to offer solutions to pressing societal and political problems. He does not conform to the traditional archetype of a philosopher; rather, he is an interdisciplinary scholar who engages with multiple disciplines. Moreover, Fromm's theories of authoritarianism and fascism, which form the basis of his critical theory, are not aimed at establishing normative standards but clearly at identifying and addressing political issues. These theories are therefore classified as theories of politics rather than political philosophies. However, the predominant focus among contemporary scholars in the humanities on Fromm's normative potential overshadows a thorough examination of his problem-solving methodologies. It is evident that the problem-solving potential inherent in Fromm's social and political theory is often overlooked, and it is frequently reduced to a rudimentary moral theory. It is important to acknowledge that social and political theorists are not synonymous with moral philosophers or moral theorists. Furthermore, the efficacy of Fromm's problem-solving approach extends beyond the realms of clinical and medical practice. Fromm's theoretical framework is inherently social and political in nature, emphasizing the collective over the individual. If we elect to concentrate on his humanistic theory, highlighting exclusively its moral value, rather than on his theories of politics, we may fail to fully comprehend the comprehensive scope of his critical theory. The pertinence of critical theory lies precisely in its capacity to facilitate diagnosis and remediation. Fromm's relevance for contemporary society is evident in his ability to provide practical and theoretical value by addressing societal problems in a diagnostic and prescriptive manner that is typically not engaged with by normative theorists or empirical scientists. This approach is distinct even from the methodologies employed in policy science and clinical fields.

## Notes

1 See, e.g., John H. Schaar, *Escape from Authority: The Perspectives of Erich Fromm* (New York: Basic Books, 1961).
2 The practical implementation of this approach may present certain challenges for academics.
3 See, e.g., Braune, *Erich Fromm's Revolutionary Hope*; 2 Durkin, *The Radical Humanism of Erich Fromm*; Wilde, *Erich Fromm and the Quest for Solidarity*.
4 James Gordon Finlayson, *Habermas: A Very Short Introduction* (Oxford: Oxford University Press, 2005), 4.

5 Takamichi Sakurai, *Political Theories of Narcissism: Towards Self-Reflections on Knowledge and Politics from the Psychoanalytic Perspectives of Erich Fromm and Fujita Shōzō* (Zurich: LIT Verlag, 2018), ch. 6.

6 See, e.g., Axel Honneth, *The Struggle for Recognition: The Moral Grammar of Social Conflicts*, Joel Anderson (Trans.) (Cambridge: Polity, 1995); Nancy Fraser and Axel Honneth, *Redistribution or Recognition? A Political-Philosophical Exchange* (London: Verso, 2003); Axel Honneth, *The I in We: Studies in the Theory of Recognition*, Joseph Ganahl (Trans.) (Cambridge: Polity, 2012).

7 See, e.g., Rainer Forst, *The Right to Justification: Elements of a Constructivist Theory of Justice*, Jeffrey Flynn (Trans.) (New York: Columbia University Press, 2012); Rainer Forst, *Justification and Critique: Towards a Critical Theory of Politics*, Ciaran Cronin (Trans.) (Cambridge: Polity, 2014); Rainer Forst, *Normativity and Power: Analyzing Social Orders of Justification*, Ciaran Cronin (Trans.) (Oxford: Oxford University Press, 2017).

# References


Adorno, Theodor W., Else Frenkel-Brunswik, Daniel J. Levinson, and R. Nevitt Sanford. *The Authoritarian Personality*. New York: Harper & Row, 1950.

Adorno, Theodor W., and Max Horkheimer. *Dialectic of Enlightenment: Philosophical Fragments*. Stanford, CA: Stanford University Press, 2002.

Agustín, Óscar García. *Left-Wing Populism: The Politics of the People*. Bingley: Emerald Group Publishing, 2020.

Altemeyer, Bob. "The Other Authoritarian Personality," in John T. Jost and Jim Sidanius (Eds.), *Political Psychology: Key Readings*. New York: Psychology Press, 2004, 85–107.

Anderson, Kevin, and Richard Quinney (Eds.). *Erich Fromm and Critical Criminology: Beyond the Punitive Society*. Urbana and Chicago: University of Illinois Press, 2000.

Atkins, Stephen E. "Introduction," in Stephen E. Atkins (Ed.), *Encyclopedia of Modern Worldwide Extremists and Extremist Groups*. Connecticut: Greenwood Press, 2004.

Bacciagaluppi, Marco. "Fromm's Views on Narcissism and the Self," in John Fiscalini and Alan. L. Grey (Eds.), *Narcissism and the Interpersonal Self*. New York: Columbia University Press, 1993, 91–106.

Bacciagaluppi, Marco. *Paradigms in Psychoanalysis: An Integration*. New York: Columbia University Press, 2012.

Bacciagaluppi, Marco, and Romano Biancoli. "Frommian Themes in a Case of Narcissistic Personality Disorder," *Contemporary Psychoanalysis*, 29, no. 3 (1993): 441–52.

Bach, Maurizio. "Fascism," in Austin Harrington, Barbara L. Marshall, and Hans-Peter Muller (Eds.), *Encyclopedia of Social Theory*. London and New York: Routledge, 2006, 192–3.

Beetham, David. *Max Weber and the Theory of Modern Politics*. Cambridge: Polity Press, 1985.

Berman, Sheri. "Populism Is Not Fascism: But It Could Be a Harbinger," *Foreign Affair*, 95, no. 6 (2016): 39–44.

von Beyme, Klaus. "Right-Wing Extremism in Post-war Europe," in Klaus von Beyme (Ed.), *Right-Wing Extremism in Western Europe*. Abingdon, Oxon: Routledge, 2013, 1–18.

Biess, Frank. *German Angst: Fear and Democracy in the Federal Republic of Germany*. New York: Oxford University Press, 2020.

Boehnke, Klaus, and Andreas Hadjar. "Authoritarianism," in Charles Spielberger (Ed.), *Encyclopedia of Applied Psychology*, Vol. 1. Oxford, Boston: Elsevier Academic Press, 2004, 151–6.

Boggs, Carl. *Fascism Old and New: American Politics at the Crossroads*. Abingdon, Oxon: Routledge, 2018.

Boucher, Geoff M. *Critical Theory and the Authoritarian Personality*. Edinburgh: Edinburgh University Press, 2025.
Braune, Joan. "Erich Fromm and Thomas Merton: Biophilia, Necrophilia, and Messianism," *Fromm Forum* (English version), 15 (2011): 43–8
Braune, Joan. *Erich Fromm's Revolutionary Hope: Prophetic Messianism as a Critical Theory of the Future*. Rotterdam: Sense Publishers, 2014.
Braune, Joan. *Understanding and Countering Fascist Movements: From Void to Hope*. Abingdon, Oxon: Routledge, 2023.
Braune, Joan, and Kieran Durkin (Eds.). *Erich Fromm's Critical Theory: Hope, Humanism, and the Future*. London: Bloomsbury Academic, 2020.
Braunthal, Gerard. *Right-Wing Extremism in Contemporary Germany*. Houndmills, Basingstoke, Hampshire: Palgrave Macmillan, 2009.
Bronner, Stephen E. "Fromm in America," in Michael Kessler and Rainer Funk (Eds.), *Erich Fromm und die Frankfurter Schule*. Tübingen: Francke Verlag, 1992, 41–59.
Brookfield, Stephen. "Overcoming Alienation as the Practice of Adult Education: The Contribution of Erich Fromm to a Critical Theory of Adult Learning and Education," *Adult Education Quarterly*, 52, no. 2 (2002): 96–111.
Brown, Wendy, Peter E. Gordon, and Max Pensky. *Authoritarianism: Three Inquiries in Critical Theory*. Chicago: Chicago University Press, 2018.
Butterwegge, Christoph, Gudrun Hentges, and Gerd Wiegel. *Rechtspopulisten im Parlament: Polemik, Agitation und Propaganda der AfD*. Frankfurt am Main: Westend Verlag, 2018.
Campbell, W. Keith, and Joshua D. Miller (Eds.). *The Handbook of Narcissism and Narcissistic Personality Disorder: Theoretical Approaches, Empirical Findings, and Treatments*. Hoboken, NJ: John Wiley & Sons, 2011.
Carroll, William K. *The Making of a Transnational Capitalist Class: Corporate Power in the 21st Century*. London: Zed Books, 2010.
Cento Bull, Anna. "Neo-Fascism," in R. J. B. Bosworth (Ed.), *The Oxford Handbook of Fascism*. Oxford: Oxford University Press, 2009, 586–605.
Charny, Israel W. *Fascism and Democracy in the Human Mind: A Bridge between Mind and Society*. Lincoln, Nebraska: University of Nebraska Press, 2006.
Cheliotis, Leonidas K. "Violence and Narcissism: A Frommian Perspective on Destructiveness under Authoritarianism," *Canadian Journal of Sociology*, 36, no. 4 (2012): 337–60.
Colliot-Thélène, Cathérine. "Populism as a Conceptual Problem," in Gregor Fitzi, Juergen Mackert, and Bryan S. Turner (Eds.), *Populism and the Crisis of Democracy: Volume 1: Concepts and Theory*. Abingdon, Oxon: Routledge, 2019, 17–26.
Connolly, William E. *Aspirational Fascism: The Struggle for Multifaceted Democracy under Trumpism*. Minneapolis: University of Minnesota Press, 2017.
Cooper, Terry D. *Paul Tillich and Psychology: Historic and Contemporary Explorations in Theology, Psychotherapy, and Ethics*. Macon, GA: Mercer University Press, 2006.
Cortina, Mauricio. "Prologue: Erich Fromm's Relevance for Our Troubled World," *Psychoanalytic Inquiry*, 44, no. 1 (2024): 1–8.
Deguchi, Takeshi. "Post-Truth Politics as a Pathology of Normalcy: Beyond Alienation and Narcissism in the Age of Globalization," *Fromm Forum*, 23 (2019): 161–8.
Durkin, Kieran. *The Radical Humanism of Erich Fromm*. New York: Palgrave Macmillan, 2014.
Ehnis, Patrick, and Katrin Voigt. "Fromm's Contribution to the Analysis and Critique of the Ongoing Rise of Right-Wing Movements," *Fromm Forum*, 23 (2019): 138–52.
Eiland, Howard, and Michael William Jennings. *Walter Benjamin: A Critical Life*. Cambridge, MA: Harvard University Press, 2014.

Essbach-Kreuzer, Uschi. „Die Theorie des Sozialcharakters in den Arbeiten von Erich Fromm," in Adelbert Reif (Hg.), *Erich Fromm: Materialien zu seinem Werk*. Wien: Europa Verlag, 1978, 299–326.

Evans, Richard I. *Dialogue with Erich Fromm*. New York: Harper and Row, 1966.

Ewen, Robert B. *An Introduction to Theories of Personality*. 7th ed. New York: Psychology Press, 2014.

Fantauzzi, Joseph, Maor Levitin, and Terry Maley (Eds.). *Erich Fromm and Left Strategy: New Paths Toward Radical Transformation*. Cham, Switzerland: Palgrave Macmillan, 2025.

Finchelstein, Federco. *From Fascism to Populism in History*. Oakland, California: University of California Press, 2017.

Finlayson, James Gordon. *Habermas: A Very Short Introduction*. Oxford: Oxford University Press, 2005.

Fiscalini, John. "Narcissism and Self-Disorder," in Marylou Lionells, John Fiscalini, Carola Mann, and Donnel B. Stern (Eds.), *Handbook of Interpersonal Psychoanalysis*. New York and London: Routledge, 2009, 333–74.

Forst, Rainer. *The Right to Justification: Elements of a Constructivist Theory of Justice*, Jeffrey Flynn (Trans). New York: Columbia University Press, 2012.

Forst, Rainer. *Justification and Critique: Towards a Critical Theory of Politics*, Ciaran Cronin (Trans). Cambridge: Polity, 2014.

Forst, Rainer. *Normativity and Power: Analyzing Social Orders of Justification*, Ciaran Cronin (Trans). Oxford: Oxford University Press, 2017.

Fozooni, Babak. *Psychology, Humour and Class: A Critique of Contemporary Psychology*. Abingdon, Oxon: Routledge, 2020.

Fraser, Nancy, and Axel Honneth. *Redistribution or Recognition? A Political-Philosophical Exchange*. London: Verso, 2003.

Frenkel-Brunswik, Else, and *The Authoritarian Personality*," in Vlad Petre Glaveanu (Ed.), *The Creativity Reader*. New York: Oxford University Press, 2019, 517–32.

Freud, Sigmund. "On Narcissism: An Introduction," in James Strachey (Ed. and Trans), *The Standard Edition of the Complete Psychological Works of Sigmund Freud*, vol. 14. London: Hogarth Press, 2001 [1953], 67–102.

Freud, Sigmund. "Introductory Lectures on Psycho-Analysis (Part III)," in James Strachey (Ed. and Trans), *The Standard Edition of the Complete Psychological Works of Sigmund Freud*, vol. 16 (1916–17). London: Hogarth Press, 2001.

Frie, Roger. *Edge of Catastrophe: Erich Fromm, Fascism, and the Holocaust*. New York: Oxford University Press, 2024.

Friedman, Lawrence Jacob. *The Lives of Erich Fromm: Love's Prophet*. New York: Columbia University Press, 2013.

Fromm, Erich. „Sozialpsychologischer Teil," in Institut für Sozialforschung (Ed.), *Studien über Autorität und Familie*.

Fromm, Erich. *Escape from Freedom*. New York: Rinehart & Company, 1941.

Fromm, Erich. "Psychoanalytic Characterology and Its Application to the Understanding of Culture," in S. Stansfeld Sargent and Marian W. Smith (Eds.), *Culture and Personality*. New York: Viking Fund, 1949, 1–12.

Fromm, Erich. *The Sane Society*. New York: Henry Holt & Company, 1956 [1955].

Fromm, Erich. *Beyond the Chains of Illusion: My Encounter with Marx and Freud*. London: Abacus, 1962.

Fromm, Erich. *The Art of Loving*. New York and Evanston: Harper & Row, 1962 [1956].

Fromm, Erich. *The Heart of Man: Its Genius for Good and Evil*. New York: Harper & Row, 1964.

Fromm, Erich. *The Crisis of Psychoanalysis: Essays on Freud, Marx, and Social Psychology*. New York: Henry Holt & Company, 1970 [1932].

Fromm, Erich. *Man for Himself: An Inquiry into the Psychology of Ethics*. London: Routledge & Kegan Paul, 1971 [1947].

Fromm, Erich. „Über Methode und Aufgaben einer analytischen Sozialpsychologie. Bemerkungen über Psychoanalyse und historischen Materialismus," in Rainer Funk (Hg.), *Erich Fromm Gesamtausgabe, Band 1: Analytische Sozialpsychologie*. Stuttgart: Deutsche Verlags-Anstalt, 1980 [1932], 37–57.

Fromm, Erich. *Greatness and Limitations of Freud's Thought*. London: Jonathan Cape, 1980 [1979].

Fromm, Erich. *The Working Class in Weimar Germany: A Psychological and Sociological Study*. Cambridge, MA: Harvard University Press, 1984.

Fromm, Erich. *Das jüdische Gesetz: Zur Soziologie des Diaspora-Judentums. Schriften aus dem Nachlaß, Band 2*, Rainer Funk (Ed.). Weinheim und Basel: Beltz Verlag, 1989 [1922].

Fromm, Erich. *The Anatomy of Human Destructiveness*. 1st ed. New York: Henry Holt & Company, 1992 [1973].

Fromm, Erich. *Man for Himself: An Inquiry into the Psychology of Ethics*. London: Routledge & Kegan Paul, 1997 [1947].

Fromm, Erich. *On Being Human*. New York: Continuum, 2005 [1997].

Fromm, Erich. *To Have or to Be?*. New York: Continuum, 2011 [1976].

Fromm, Erich. *Marx's Concept of Man*. London: Bloomsbury Academic, 2013 [1961].

Fuchs, Christian. *Digital Demagogue: Authoritarian Capitalism in the Age of Trump and Twitter*. London: Pluto Press, 2018.

Fuchs, Christian. *Nationalism on the Internet: Critical Theory and Ideology in the Age of Social Media and Fake News*. Abingdon, Oxon: Routledge, 2019.

Fuchs, Christian. *Digital Fascism: Media, Communication and Society Volume Four*. Abingdon, Oxon: Routledge, 2022.

Funk, Rainer. "Fromm's Method of Social Psychology," Lecture at the American Academy of Psychoanalysis, 34th Winter Meeting, Hilton Palacio del Rio, San Antonio, Texas, US, December 8, 1990. http://opus4.kobv.de/opus4Fromm/files /9899/Funk_R_1990e.pdf.1990.

Funk, Rainer. „Narzissmus und Gewalttätigkeit gegen Fremdes," in Internationale Erich-Fromm-Gesellschaft (Ed.), *Jahrbuch der Internationalen Erich-Fromm-Gesellschaft, vol. 5: Vom Umgang mit dem Fremden (Dealing with the Alien)*. Münster: LIT Verlag, 1993, 45–60.

Funk, Rainer. „Egoismus als Selbstsucht und Narzissmus: Überlegungen in Anschluss an Erich Fromm," in Thomas Leon Heck (Ed.), *Das Prinzip Egoismus*. Tübingen: Nous Verlag, 1994, 353–66.

Funk, Rainer. "Erich Fromm's Concept of Social Character and Its Relevance for Clinical Practice," in Mauricio Cortina and Michael Maccoby (Eds.), *A Prophetic Analyst: Erich Fromm's Contribution to Psychoanalysis*. Northvale and London: Jason Aronson, 1996, 341–60.

Funk, Rainer. "The Continuing Relevance of Erich Fromm," *Fromm Forum* (English edn.), 4 (2000): 9–14.

Funk, Rainer. *Das Leben selbst ist eine Kunst. Einführung in Leben und Werk von Erich Fromm*, Neuausgabe. Freiburg: Herder, 2018.

Funk, Rainer. "Erich Fromm: Bringing Psychoanalysis and Sociology Together," *Fromm Forum* (English edn.), 23 (2019): 9–23.

Funk, Rainer, and Thomas Kühn. "Introduction," *Fromm Forum* (English edn.), 23 (2019): 5–8.

Funk, Rainer, and Neil McLaughlin. "Introduction," in Funk and McLaughlin (Eds.), *Towards a Human Science: The Relevance of Erich Fromm for Today*. Gießen: Psychosozial-Verlag, 2015.

Geyer, R. Felix, and David R. Schweitzer (Eds.). *Theories of Alienation: Critical Perspectives in Philosophy and the Social Sciences*. Cham, Switzerland: Springer, 2012 [1976].

Ginzel, Günther B. *Hitlers (Ur)enkel: Neo-Nazis, Ihre Ideologien und Aktionen*. Düsseldorf: Droste, 1981.

Giroux, Henry A. *American Nightmare: Facing the Challenge of Fascism*. San Francisco: City Lights Books, 2018.

Gottfried, Shelly. *Contemporary Oligarchies in Developed Democracies*. Cham, Switzerland: Palgrave Macmillan, 2019.

Gregor, A. James. *Interpretations of Fascism*. Abingdon, Oxon: Routledge, 2017.

Grey, Alan. "Society as Destiny: Fromm's Concept of Social Character," *Contemporary Psychoanalysis*, 28, no. 2 (1992): 344–63.

Griffin, Roger. "The 'Post-Fascism' of the Alleanza Nazionale: A case Study in Ideological Morphology," *Journal of Political Ideologies*, 1, no. 2 (1996): 123–45.

Griffin, Roger. *A Fascist Century: Essays by Roger Griffin*. Houndmills, Basingstoke, Hampshire: Palgrave Macmillan, 2008.

Griffin, Roger. "Studying Fascism in a Postfascist Age: From New Consensus to New Wave?" *Fascism: Journal of Comparative Fascist Studies*, 1 (2012): 1–17.

Grist, Leighton. *Fascism and Millennial American Cinema*. London: Palgrave Macmillan, 2018.

Hathaway, Terry. "Neoliberalism as Corporate Power," *Competition & Change*, 24, no. 3–4 (2020): 315–37.

Henning, Christoph. *Theories of Alienation: From Rousseau to the Present*. Abingdon, Oxon: Routledge, 2024.

Herman Brinks, Jan. *Children of a New Fatherland: Germany's Post-War Right-Wing Politics*. London: I.B. Tauris, 2000.

Herman Brinks, Jan. "Germany's New Right," in Jan Herman Brinks, Stella Rock, and Edward Timms (Eds.), *Nationalist Myths and Modern Media: Contested Identities in the Age of Globalization*. London: I.B. Tauris, 2006, 125–38.

Hermansson, Patrik, David Lawrence, Joe Mulhall, and Simon Murdoch. *The International Alt-Right: Fascism for the 21st Century?* Abingdon, Oxon: Routledge, 2020.

Hewer, Christopher J., and Evanthia Lyons (Eds.). *Political Psychology: A Social Psychological Approach*. Hoboken, NJ: Wiley, 2018.

Hawley, George. *The Alt-Right*. New York: Oxford University Press, 2019.

Hofstede, Geert. *Culture's Consequences: International Differences in Work-Related Values*. Newbury Park, CA: Sage, 1980.

Honneth, Axel. *The Struggle for Recognition: The Moral Grammar of Social Conflicts*, Joel Anderson (Trans). Cambridge: Polity, 1995.

Honneth, Axel. *The I in We: Studies in the Theory of Recognition*, Joseph Ganahl (Trans). Cambridge: Polity, 2012.

Horkheimer, Max. "The Social Function of Philosophy," in M. Horkheimer (Ed.), *Critical Theory: Selected Essays*. New York: Continuum, 2002, 253–72.

Horkheimer, Max. "Traditional and Critical Theory," in Max Horkheimer (Ed.), *Critical Theory: Selected Essays*. New York: Continuum, 2002 [1972], 188–243.

Horney Eckardt, Marianne. "Fromm's Humanistic Ethics and the Role of the Prophet," in Mauricio Cortina and Michael Maccoby (Eds.), *A Prophetic Analyst: Erich Fromm's Contribution to Psychoanalysis*. Northvale and London: Jason Aronson, 1996, 151–66.

Hough, Dan, and Dan Keith. "The German Left Party: A Case of Pragmatic Populism," in Giorgos Katsambekis and Alexandros Kioupkiolis (Eds.), *The Populist Radical Left in Europe*. Abingdon, Oxon: Routledge, 2019.

Ingleby, David. "Introduction to the Second Edition of *The Same Society*," in Erich Fromm (Ed.), *The Sane Society*. Abingdon, Oxon: Routledge: 2002 [1955], xvi–Iv.
Institut für Sozialforschung (Ed.). *Studien über Autorität und Familie*. Paris: Alcan, 1936.
Jäger, Siegfried. "Political Discourse: The Language of Right and Left in Germany," in Patrick Stevenson (Ed.), *The German Language and the Real World: Sociolinguistic, Cultural, and Pragmatic Perspectives on Contemporary German*, revised ed. Oxford: Clarendon Press, 1997, 233–57.
Jimenez, Luis. "Revisiting Fromm's Concept of Social Character and Social Change: An Example from De-Industrialized Working Class Communities in the UK," *Fromm Forum*, 23 (2019): 182–98.
Kautzer, Chad. "Marx's Influence on the Early Frankfurt School," in Michael J. Thompson (Ed.), *The Palgrave Handbook of Critical Theory*. New York: Palgrave Macmillan, 2017, 43–66.
Kaya, Ayhan. *Populism and Heritage in Europe: Lost in Diversity and Unity*. Abingdon, Oxon: Routledge, 2020.
Kellner, Douglas. *American Nightmare: Donald Trump, Media Spectacle, and Authoritarian Populism*. Rotterdam: Sense Publishers, 2016.
Kellner, Douglas. "Donald Trump, Media Spectacle, and Authoritarian Populism," *Fast Capitalism*, 14, no. 1 (2017): 75–87.
Kellner, Douglas. "Donald Trump as Authoritarian Populist: A Frommian Analysis," in Jeremiah Morelock (Ed.), *Critical Theory and Authoritarian Populism*. London: University of Westminster Press, 2018, 71–82.
Kitagawa, Takayoshi, and Takashi Miyajima (Eds.). *Nijusseiki shakaigaku riron no tanjō* [The Birth of Twenty-Century Sociological Theory]. Tokyo: Yūshindō, 1996.
Kitchen, Martin. *Fascism*. Houndmills, Basingstoke, Hampshire: Macmillan, 1976.
Koch, József. "Erich Fromm's Humanistic View of Man and Our Divided World," Paper for the International Erich Fromm Society's seminar on Character Structure and Society, Janus Pannonius University, Hungary, August 24–26, 1990. http://opus4.kobv.de/opus4-Fromm/files/13699/Koch_J_1990c.pdf.
Laqueur, Walter (Ed.). *Fascism: A Reader's Guide: Analyses, Interpretations, Bibliography*. Berkeley and Los Angeles: University of California Press, 1976.
Lesser, Ruth. "Erich Fromm and the Psychoanalysis of the Social Unconscious," *Fromm Forum* (English version), 6 (2002): 23–24.
Levitsky, Steven, and Lucan A. Way. *Competitive Authoritarianism Hybrid Regimes after the Cold War*. New York: Cambridge University Press, 2010.
Levy, Kenneth, William D. Ellison, and Joseph S. Reynoso. "A Historical Review of Narcissism and Narcissistic Personality," in W. Keith Campbell and Joshua D. Miller (Eds.), *The Handbook of Narcissism and Narcissistic Personality Disorder: Theoretical Approaches, Empirical Findings, and Treatments*. Hoboken, NJ: John Wiley & Sons, 2011, 3–13.
Lewis, Rand C. *The Neo-Nazis and German Unification*. Westport, Connecticut and London: Praeger, 1996.
Linz, Juan J. "An Authoritarian Regime: The Case of Spain," in Erik Allardt and Yrjö Littunen (Eds.), *Cleavages, Ideologies, and Party Systems: Contributions to Comparative Political Sociology*. Helsinki: Academic Bookstore, 1964, 291–341.
Lio, Enzo. "Alienation as a Central Concept in Marxist and Frommian Humanism," Presentation at a German-Italian Seminar about Die Marx Rezeption Erich Fromms, Bologna, Italy, February 17–19, 1989. http://www.frommgesellschaft.eu/images/pdf–Dateien/Lio_E_1989b.pdf.
Loyal, Steven, and Sinisa Malesevic. *Contemporary Sociological Theory*. London: Sage, 2020.

Lundskow, George. *The Sociology of Religion: A Substantive and Transdisciplinary Approach*. London: Sage, 2008.
Maccoby, Michael. "Toward a Science of Social Character," *International Forum of Psychoanalysis*, 11, no. 1 (2002): 33–44.
Maccoby, Michael, and Neil McLaughlin, "Sociopsychoanalysis and Radical Humanism: A Fromm-Bourdieu Synthesis," *Fromm Forum* (English edn.), 23 (2019): 45–57.
Mammone, Andrea, Emmanuel Godin, and Brian Jenkins, "Introduction," in Andrea Mammone, Emmanuel Godin, and Brian Jenkins (Eds.), *Varieties of Right-Wing Extremism in Europe*. Abingdon, Oxon: Routledge, 2013, 1–15.
Marcuse, Herbert. *From the New Left to the Next Left*. Lawrence, KS: University Press of Kansas, 1994.
Marmor, Judd. *Modern Psychoanalysis: New Directions and Perspectives*. New York: Basic Books, 1968.
Marx, Karl. *Capital, vol. 1: A Critique of Political Economy*, Ben Fowkes (Trans). London: Penguin Classics, 1992 [1867].
Marx, Karl. *Economic and Philosophical Manuscripts*, Thomas B. Bottomore (Trans), in Erich Fromm (Ed.), *Marx's Concept of Man*. London: Bloomsbury Academic, 2013 [1844].
McLaughlin, Neil. "Nazism, Nationalism, and the Sociology of Emotions: *Escape from Freedom* Revisited," *Sociological Theory*, 14, no. 3 (1996): 241–61.
McLaughlin, Neil. "How to Become a Forgotten Intellectual: Intellectual Movements and the Rise and Fall of Erich Fromm," *Sociological Forum*, 13 (1998): 215–46.
McLaughlin, Neil. "Who Killed off Fromm's Reputation in North America? Russell Jacoby's Social Amnesia and the Forgetting of a Public Intellectual," *Fromm Forum* (English edn.), 21 (2017): 7–21.
McLaughlin, Neil. *Erich Fromm and Global Public Sociology*. Bristol: Bristol University Press, 2021.
Merrotsy, Peter. "Authoritarian Personality," in Fathali M. Moghaddam (Ed.), *The SAGE Encyclopedia of Political Behavior*. London: Sage, 2017, 45–47.
Millán, Salvador. "The Third World and the Social Character," in International Erich Fromm Society (Ed.), *Wissenschaft vom Menschen/Science of Man*, vol. 3. Münster: LIT Verlag, 1992, 57–67.
Millán, Salvador. "The Social Dimensions of Transference," Paper for the Erich Fromm International Symposium, Washington, DC, 1–7, May 8, 1994. http://opus4.kobv.de/opus4-Fromm/files/16525/Millan_S_1992.pdf.
Minkenburg, Michael. "The New Radical Right in the Political Process: Interaction Effects in France and Germany," in Martin Schain, Patrick Hossay, and Aristide R. Zolberg (Ed.), *Shadows Over Europe: The Development and Impact of the Extreme Right in Western Europe*. New York: Palgrave Macmillan, 2002, 245–68.
Morelock, Jeremiah (Ed.). *Critical Theory and Authoritarian Populism*. London: University of Westminster Press, 2018.
Morelock, Jeremiah (Ed.). *How to Critique Authoritarian Populism: Methodologies of the Frankfurt School*. Leiden and Boston: Brill, 2021.
Mudde, Cas, and Cristóbal Rovira Kaltwasser. *Populism: A Very Short Introduction*. New York: Oxford University Press, 2017.
Neumann, Klaus. "Inter-War Germany and the Corporatist Wave, 1918–1939," in Antonio Costa Pinto (Ed.), *Corporatism and Fascism: The Corporatist Wave in Europe*. Abingdon, Oxon: Routledge, 2017, 124–43.
Norris, Pippa, and Ronald Inglehart. *Cultural Backlash: Trump, Brexit, and Authoritarian Populism*. Cambridge: Cambridge University Press, 2019.
Ortmeyer, Dale H. "Clinical Relevance of Social Character and Social Unconscious," *International Forum of Psychoanalysis*, 11, no. 1 (2002): 4–9.

Pabst, Adrian. *The Demons of Liberal Democracy*. Cambridge: Polity, 2019.

Paić, Žarko. *Neoliberalism, Oligarchy and Politics of the Event: At the Edge of Chaos*. Newcastle upon Tyne: Cambridge Scholars Publishing, 2020.

Panfilova, Tatiana. "Social Character and Social Unconscious: Erich Fromm's Discovery and the Problems of Today," in Funk and McLaughlin (Eds.), *Towards a Human Science*. 201–7.

Passmore, Kevin. *Fascism: A Very Short Introduction*. Oxford: Oxford University Press, 2014 [2002].

Pausch, Markus. *Demokratie als Revolte: Zwischen Alltagsdiktatur und Globalisierung*. Baden-Baden: Nomos, 2017.

Pausch, Markus. "Democracy Needs Rebellion: A Democratic Theory Inspired by Albert Camus," *Theoria: A Journal of Social and Political Theory*, 66, no. 161 (2019): 91–107.

Pegida. "28. Jahrestag des Mauerfalls," *Pegida*, November 9, 2017. https://www.pegida.de/news/28-jahrestag-des-mauerfalls.html.

Peters, Michael A. "'The Fascism in Our Heads': Reich, Fromm, Foucault, Deleuze and Guattari – The Social Pathology of Fascism in the 21st Century," *Educational Philosophy and Theory*, 54, no. 9 (2020): 1276–84.

Petry, Frauke. "Wir sind der Stachel im Fleisch," Philip Eppelsheim (Intvw.), *Frankfurter Allgemeine Woche*, 20 (2018): 27–29.

Pickering, Michael, and Thomas Kehoe (Eds.). *Fear in the German-Speaking World, 1600-2000*. New York: Bloomsbury.

Plehwe, Dieter, Bernhard J. A. Walpen, and Gisela Neunhöffer. *Neoliberal Hegemony: A Global Critique*. Abingdon, Oxon: Routledge, 2006.

Rabinbach, Anson. "Between Apocalypse and Enlightenment: Benjamin, Bloch and Modern German Jewish Messianism," in Peter Osborne (Ed.), *Walter Benjamin: Critical Evaluations in Cultural Theory*, Vol. 3. Abingdon, Oxon: Routledge, 2005, 116–61.

Rattray, Mary. "Erich Fromm: A Twentieth Century Prophet?". M.Th. Thesis, University of Glasgow, 1995.

Reid, Shannon.E., and Matthew Valasik. *Alt-Right Gangs: A Hazy Shade of White*. Oakland, California: University of California Press, 2020.

Roberts, David D. *Fascist Interactions: Proposals for a New Approach to Fascism and Its Era, 1919–1945*. New York and Oxford: Berghahn, 2016.

Robinson. William I. *A Theory of Global Capitalism: Production, Class, and State in a Transnational World*. Baltimore, MD: Johns Hopkins University Press, 2004.

Robinson, William I. *Global Capitalism and the Crisis of Humanity*. New York: Cambridge University Press, 2014.

Robinson, William I., and Jeb Sprague. "The Transnational Capitalist Class," in Mark Juergensmeyer, Saskia Sassen, Manfred B. Steger, and Victor Faessel (Eds.), *The Oxford handbook of Global Studies*. New York: Oxford University Press, 2018, 309–27.

Ronningstam, Elsa F. *Identifying and Understanding the Narcissistic Personality*. New York: Oxford University Press, 2005.

Rudnytsky, Peter L. "The Social Determinants of Psychoanalytic Therapy: Fromm's Anti-Authoritarian 'Calling Card'," *Psychoanalytic Inquiry*, 44, no. 1 (2024): 9–14.

Ruzza, Carlo, and Stefano Fella. *Re-Inventing the Italian Right: Territorial Politics, Populism and 'Post-Fascism'*. Abingdon, Oxon: Routledge, 2009.

Sakurai, Takamichi. *Political Theories of Narcissism: Towards Self-Reflection on Knowledge and Politics from the Psychoanalytic Perspectives of Erich Fromm and Fujita Shōzō (Politikwissenschaft, Band 212)*. Zurich: LIT Verlag, 2018.

Sakurai, Takamichi. "The Socio-Psychological Base of Contemporary Fascism in the World of Liberal Democracy: The Theoretical Scope of Erich Fromm's Socio-Pathological Theory of Alienation," *Fromm Forum* (English edn.), 22 (2018): 143–55.

Sakurai, Takamichi. "Minshushugi ni okeru media to rondan: Doitsu no nyūsu magajin ni miru kami-baitai no gendaiteki jōken" (The Functions of Media and Opinion Leaders in Contemporary Democracy: The Present State of Paper-Based Opinion Magazines, as Evidenced by German News Magazines), *Jōkyō* (fifth ed.), 1, no. 1 (2018): 8–22.

Sakurai, Takamichi. "A Frommian Perspective on the Socio-Psychological Structure of Post-Fascism in Liberal Democracies," *Distinktion: Journal of Social Theory*, 21, no. 2 (2020): 178–94.

Sakurai, Takamichi. "The Socio-Theoretical Relevance of Erich Fromm's Psychoanalytic Conception of Narcissism: Towards a Frommian Critical Social Theory of Narcissism," *Theoria: A Journal of Social and Political Theory*, 68, no. 166 (2021): 1–30.

Sakurai, Takamichi. "Aspirational Fascism versus Postfascism: A Conceptual History of a Far-Right Politics," *History of European Ideas*, 48, no. 5 (2022): 650–60.

Sakurai, Takamichi. "The Authoritarian Orientation in Liberal Democracies: Labour Market and Workplace Authoritarianism," *Constellations*, 32, no. 1 (2025): 59–68.

Sayers, Sean. *Marx and Alienation: Essays on Hegelian Themes*. Basingstoke and New York: Palgrave Macmillan, 2011.

Schaar, John H. *Escape from Authority: The Perspectives of Erich Fromm*. New York: Basic Books, 1961.

Schacht, Richard. *The Future of Alienation*. Urbana and Chicago: University of Illinois Press, 1994.

Schacht, Richard. *Alienation*. London: Psychology Press, 2015 [1970].

Sklair, Leslie. *The Transnational Capitalist Class*. Oxford: Blackwell, 2011.

Smith, Mark K. "Erich Fromm: Alienation, Being and Education," in *The Encyclopedia of Informal Education*, 2002. http://www.infed.org/thinkers/fromm.htm.

Stanley, Jason. *How Fascism Works: The Politics of US and Them*. New York: Random House, 2018.

Sterphone, Joseph. "'Mut zu Deutschland!' On the populist nationalism of the Alternative für Deutschland," in Fernando López-Alves and Diane E. Johnson (Eds.), *Populist Nationalism in Europe and the Americas*. New York: Routledge, 2019, 99–115.

Tamás, Gáspár Miklós. "On Post-Fascism: The Degradation of Universal Citizenship," *Boston Review: A Political and Literary Forum*, June 1, 2000. http://bostonreview.net/world/g-m-tamas-post-fascism.

Tamás, Gáspár Miklós. "What Is Post-Fascism?," *openDemocracy*. September 31, 2001. https://www.opendemocracy.net/en/article_306jsp.

Thompson, Michael J. "Normative Humanism and Redemptive Critique: Knowledge and Judgement in Erich Fromm's Social Theory," in Seyed Javad Miri, Robert Lake, and Tricia M. Kress (Eds.), *Reclaiming the Sane Society: Essays on Erich Fromm's Thought*. Rotterdam: Sense Publishers, 2014, 37–58.

Thomson, Annette. *Erich Fromm: Shaper of the Human Condition*. London: Palgrave Macmillan, 2009.

Thorpe, Charles. *Necroculture*. New York: Palgrave Macmillan, 2016.

Thorpe, Charles. "Escape from Reflexivity: Fromm and Giddens on Individualism, Anxiety, and Authoritarianism," in Joan Braune and Kieran Durkin (Eds.), *Erich Fromm's Critical Theory: Hope, Humanism, and the Future*. London: Bloomsbury Academic, 2020.

Traverso, Enzo. *The New Faces of Fascism: Populism and the Far Right*, David Broder (Trans). London: Verso, 2019.
Tummers, Lars. *Policy Alienation and the Power of Professionals: Confronting New Policies*. Northampton: Edward Elgar, 2013.
Tyner, James A. *The Alienated Subject: On the Capacity to Hurt*. Minneapolis, MN: University of Minnesota Press, 2022.
Vadolas, Antonios. *Perversions of Fascism*. London: Karnac Books, 2009.
Vorländer, Hans, Maik Herold, and Steven Schäller. *PEGIDA and New Right-Wing Populism in Germany*. Cham, Switzerland: Palgrave Macmillan, 2018.
Weber, Max. *Gesammelte Politische Schriften*. Tübingen: J.C.B. Mohr, 1988.
Weidel, Alice. *Widerworte: Gedanken über Deutschland*. Kulmbach: Plassen Verlag, 2019.
Whitebook, Joel. "Fantasy and Critique: Some Thoughts on Freud and the Frankfurt School," in David M. Rasmusssen (Ed.), *The Handbook of Critical Theory*. Oxford: Blackwell, 1996, 287–304.
Whittam, John. *Fascist Italy*. Manchester and New York: Manchester University Press, 1995.
Wiarda, Howard J. *Corporatism and Comparative Politics: The Other Great 'Ism'*. Abingdon, Oxon: Routledge, 2015 [1997].
Wilde, Lawrence. *Erich Fromm and the Quest for Solidarity*. Houndmills, Basingstoke, Hampshire: Palgrave Macmillan, 2004.
Wilson, Carter A. *Trumpism: Race, Class, Populism, and Public Policy*. Lexington, MA: Lexington Books, 2021.
Wozniak, John F. "Alienation and Crime: Lessons from Erich Fromm," in Kevin Anderson and Richard Quinney (Eds.), *Erich Fromm and Critical Criminology: Beyond the Punitive Society*. Urbana and Chicago: University of Illinois Press, 2000, 43–58.
Xirau, Ramon. "Erich Fromm: What Is Man's Struggle?" in Bernard Landis and Edward S. Tauber (Eds.), *In the Name of Life: Essays in Honor of Erich Fromm*. New York: Holt, Rinehart & Winston, 1971, 150–60.
Zakai, Avihu. *Jewish Exiles' Psychological Interpretations of Nazism*. Cham, Switzerland: Palgrave Macmillan, 2020.

# Index

Note: Page numbers in italics refer to tables and a figure, while 'n' denotes note numbers.

For Product Safety Concerns and Information please contact our EU representative GPSR@taylorandfrancis.com Taylor & Francis Verlag GmbH, Kaufingerstraße 24, 80331 München, Germany